STUDENT STUDY GUIDE TO ACCOMPANY

Pediatric Nursing

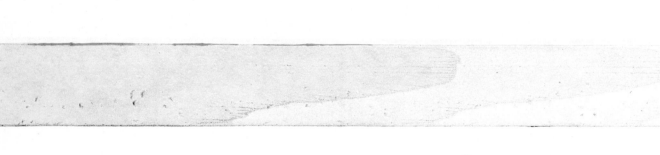

Pediatric Nursing
Caring for Children and Their Families

THIRD EDITION

Nicki L. Potts, RN, PhD

Former Instructor, College of Nursing
University of New Mexico
Albuquerque, New Mexico
Former Assistant Professor, School of Nursing
University of Texas, Austin
Austin, Texas

Barbara L. Mandleco, RN, PhD

Professor
College of Nursing
Brigham Young University
Provo, Utah

Prepared by

Valerie O'Toole Baker, ACNS, BC

Assistant Professor
Villa Maria School of Nursing
Gannon University
Erie, Pennsylvania

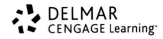

Australia • Brazil • Japan • Korea • Mexico • Singapore • Spain • United Kingdom • United States

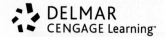

Pediatric Nursing: Caring for Children and Their Families, Third Edition
Nicki L. Potts and Barbara L. Mandleco

Vice President, Career and Professional Editorial: Dave Garza

Director of Learning Solutions: Matthew Kane

Senior Acquisitions Editor: Maureen Rosener

Managing Editor: Marah Bellegarde

Senior Product Manager: Elisabeth F. Williams

Editorial Assistant: Samantha Miller

Content Project Manager: Anne Sherman

Production Technology Analyst: Patti Allen

Vice President, Career and Professional Marketing: Jennifer McAvey

Marketing Director: Wendy Mapstone

Marketing Manager: Michelle McTighe

Marketing Coordinator: Scott Chrysler

Production Director: Carolyn Miller

Production Manager: Andrew Crouth

Senior Art Director: Jack Pendleton

Library of Congress Control Number: 2010925842

ISBN-13: 978-1-4354-8670-6

ISBN-10: 1-4354-8670-6

Delmar
Executive Woods
5 Maxwell Drive
Clifton Park, NY 12065
USA

Cengage Learning is a leading provider of customized learning solutions with office locations around the globe, including Singapore, the United Kingdom, Australia, Mexico, Brazil, and Japan. Locate your local office at **www.cengage.com/global**

Cengage Learning products are represented in Canada by Nelson Education, Ltd.

To learn more about Delmar, visit **www.cengage.com/delmar**

Purchase any of our products at your local bookstore or at our preferred online store **www.cengagebrain.com**

Notice to the Reader

Publisher does not warrant or guarantee any of the products described herein or perform any independent analysis in connection with any of the product information contained herein. Publisher does not assume, and expressly disclaims, any obligation to obtain and include information other than that provided to it by the manufacturer. The reader is expressly warned to consider and adopt all safety precautions that might be indicated by the activities described herein and to avoid all potential hazards. By following the instructions contained herein, the reader willingly assumes all risks in connection with such instructions. The publisher makes no representations or warranties of any kind, including but not limited to, the warranties of fitness for particular purpose or merchantability, nor are any such representations implied with respect to the material set forth herein, and the publisher takes no responsibility with respect to such material. The publisher shall not be liable for any special, consequential, or exemplary damages resulting, in whole or part, from the readers' use of, or reliance upon, this material.

Printed in the United States of America
2 3 4 5 6   19 18 17 16 15

Contents

Preface

The purpose of the *Student Study Guide to Accompany Pediatric Nursing: Caring for Children and Their Families,* Third Edition, is to help you learn, absorb, and retain difficult and often unfamiliar concepts in pediatric nursing. This study guide will help reinforce the major concepts as you review the central facts of each textbook chapter, as well as to develop the knowledge and skills you will need to succeed as a nurse in any health care setting.

Each chapter of the study guide contains learning exercises that draw on key ideas from the textbook. The activities include true or false, fill in the blank, matching, and multiple choice questions. New to this edition are multiple response questions, formatted according to the revised test plan for the NCLEX-RN exam; and matching questions for every chapter. In addition, each chapter features a case study or pediatric nursing scenario with critical thinking questions that test your understanding and application of important concepts.

CHAPTER 1

Overview of Pediatric Nursing

True or False

1. Child health care has changed from a disease prevention and health promotion model to strictly a curative approach.

   ❑ True ❑ False

2. The fastest-growing segment of the homeless population consists of families with children.

   ❑ True ❑ False

3. Youth violence is the second leading cause of death in U.S. citizens ages 10 to 24.

   ❑ True ❑ False

4. Because *Healthy People* emphasizes health promotion and prevention, almost all of it pertains to nursing.

   ❑ True ❑ False

5. Among children under 1 year of age, suffocation is the leading cause of unintentional injury-related death.

   ❑ True ❑ False

6. The focus of pediatric nursing is on the family as well as the child.

   ❑ True ❑ False

7. Agriculture surpasses mining and construction as the most hazardous occupation in the U.S.

   ❑ True ❑ False

Fill in the Blank

1. The risk of poverty in single-parent households is high for several reasons, including _____, _____, and _____.

2. The most common physical health problems of homeless children include _____, _____, and _____.

3. The leading health indicators of *Healthy People 2010* are _____, _____, _____, _____, _____, _____, _____, _____, and _____.

4. A low birth-weight infant is considered to weigh less than _____ at birth.

5. The key approaches to injury prevention are _____, _____, and _____.

6. Children of migrant families are at risk for two major hazards related to the agriculture industry. They include _____ and _____.

7. The philosophy of providing care that minimizes or eliminates physical and psychological distress for children and their families in the health care environment is called _____.

Matching

____ 1. cognitive learning

____ 2. advocate

____ 3. affective learning

a. involves sharing feelings and ideas

b. pleads for and assists others to make informed decisions

c. involves describing or explaining

Multiple Choice

1. When teaching adolescents, the nurse utilizes knowledge of cognitive development appropriate to this age group. Which of the following is the best technique for the nurse to incorporate in the health education of adolescents?

   a. Adolescents learn best when they see an immediate personal benefit.
   b. Adolescents have short attention spans and learn best in brief stages.
   c. Allow the adolescent to explore the environment and handle equipment.
   d. Adolescents like to imitate others, so imitation would be an appropriate method of teaching this age group.

2. The nurse teaches a 10-year-old how to administer insulin. Which learning domain is the nurse using in the teaching plan?

    a. affective learning
    b. cognitive learning
    c. psychomotor learning
    d. memorized learning

3. When following the differentiated practice model, an associate degree nurse, according to experience, competence, and education, would function in which environment?

    a. a variety of settings using independent nursing judgments based on specialized knowledge, research, and theory
    b. an ambulatory care setting focused on disease prevention, minor disease management, and well children
    c. a structured or unstructured setting with responsibilities to integrate client care from preadmission to postdischarge using independent nursing judgment
    d. a structured setting in which procedures and policies are established and followed

Multiple Response

1. In caring for a 3-year-old child who has fallen and requires sutures on his or her face, the nurse includes which of the following interventions in the provision of atraumatic care? Select all that apply.

    a. Control pain by administering analgesics freely.
    b. Prepare the child prior to every procedure using age-appropriate explanations.
    c. Use EMLA cream at least 10 minutes prior to blood draws, insertion of IV needles, and injections.
    d. Allow caregivers to be involved and physically present as much as possible.
    e. Perform painful procedures when the child falls asleep.
    f. Encourage the caregivers to leave the room when the suturing takes place.

2. Pediatric nurses act as advocates for the child and family in which of the following ways? Select all that apply.

   a. making decisions for the child and family based on what the nurse feels is in their best interest
   b. informing children and families of their rights and options
   c. providing privacy
   d. providing information about research
   e. providing information about experimental protocols
   f. providing information about alternative treatments

3. Which of the following statements about standards of care and standards of professional practice are true? Select all that apply.

   a. Standards of care are the accepted action expected of an individual with a certain skill or knowledge level.
   b. They are considered the maximal level of functioning and what a reasonable and prudent person would do in a similar situation.
   c. Standards are a tool for determining if the care provided was adequate or negligent.
   d. Professional standards are derived from regulatory agencies.
   e. Professional standards are derived from nursing practice acts.
   f. Professional standards are derived from state or federal law.

Critical Thinking/Case Study

The recent increase and public awareness of juvenile violence has many individuals concerned about the well-being of their children. The nurse has been asked to provide a series of educational programs for caregivers focused on the prevention of juvenile violence.

1. Summarize statistics about the state of juvenile violence in the United States.

   _____

   _____

   _____

2. How would the implementation of gun laws affect juvenile violence?

   _____

   _____

   _____

3. Provide a teaching plan for the family on firearm injury prevention.

   _____

   _____

   _____

4. What role in the school and community can caregivers take to affect juvenile violence?

   _____

   _____

   _____

5. In what ways can the nurse act as an advocate for children and families to affect juvenile violence?

   _____

   _____

   _____

CHAPTER 2

Legal and Ethical Issues

True or False

1. Health care is often controlled by federal laws and regulations and does not vary from state to state.

   ❏ True   ❏ False

2. Pediatric clients are entitled to informed consent.

   ❏ True   ❏ False

3. The age of majority is the age, determined by state law, at which a person is considered to have all the legal rights and responsibilities of an adult.

   ❏ True   ❏ False

4. In most states, care for pregnancy or sexually transmitted infection requires parental consent and notification.

   ❏ True   ❏ False

5. After divorce, the ability to consent for medical care of a child rests with the mother.

   ❏ True   ❏ False

6. Only persons 18 years of age and older are protected by the Health Insurance Portability and Accountability Act (HIPAA).

   ❏ True   ❏ False

7. A situation that increases the risk for malpractice or negligence in caring for pediatric clients is medication errors.

   ❏ True   ❏ False

8. The role of an ethics committee is to provide the final decision when an ethical conflict arises.

   ❏ True   ❏ False

9. When death is due to homicide, suicide, mysterious circumstances, or, in some cases, accident, an autopsy will be performed regardless of the wishes of the parents or legal guardians.

   ❏ True   ❏ False

10. Most health care facilities will provide care to a minor in an emergency situation if informed consent cannot be obtained.

    ❏ True   ❏ False

Fill in the Blank

1. _____ is the duty of a health care provider to discuss the risks and benefits of a treatment or procedure with a client prior to giving care.

2. _____ means the pediatric client has been informed about what will happen during the treatment or procedure and is willing to permit a health care provider to perform the care.

3. A(n) _____ is defined as a person who has not yet reached the age when she or he is considered to have the rights and responsibilities of an adult.

4. A(n) _____ is performed for the purpose of collecting medical evidence when the health care provider suspects the client may be a victim of a crime.

5. _____ is the application of ethics into the lives of individuals via the health care system.

6. _____ is the legal recognition that a minor lives independently and is now responsible for his or her own support and decision making.

7. Allowing a child to die by withdrawing treatment could be deemed as the use of _____.

8. The _____ is the age, determined by state law, at which a person is considered to have all the legal rights and responsibilities of an adult.

Matching

_____ 1. negligence

_____ 2. value

_____ 3. malpractice

_____ 4. plaintiff

_____ 5. morality

_____ 6. veracity

_____ 7. justice

_____ 8. beneficence

a. constructs used to give meaning to our lives

b. behavior in accordance with custom or tradition that usually reflects personal or religious beliefs

c. in a case of malpractice, the person making the claim

d. professional negligence

e. person owes a duty to another and, through failure to fulfill that duty, causes harm

f. "to do good"

g. the provision of fair and equitable care regardless of gender, culture, ethnicity, religious beliefs and practices, educational levels, or socioeconomic status

h. clear and open communication between providers and parents, and health care is transparent

Multiple Choice

1. If a health care provider treats a client without proper consent, she may be charged with which one of the following and held liable for any damages?

   a. battery
   b. kidnapping
   c. assault
   d. malpractice

2. An 8-year-old child is admitted to the health care facility for regulation of insulin therapy for his unstable diabetes mellitus. The nurse, upon assessment of the child, finds multiple snack and candy wrappers in the room as well as a large bag of open candy. When the nurse questions the child about these items, the child replies, "I got this stuff from the machine. I can do what I want; don't tell me what to do!" Which of the following would be the best documentation the nurse could make for this situation?

   a. The child is appropriately following Erickson's developmental stage of autonomy.
   b. Multiple candy and snack wrappers were found in the room along with an open bag of candy. The child stated, "I got this stuff from the machine. I can do what I want; don't tell me what to do!"
   c. Inappropriate compliance with diabetic plan of care.
   d. This child is very angry and noncompliant with the plan of care. A psychiatric consult should be made.

3. A health care organization rations health care services to developmentally disabled children. Their rationale is that their actions would serve the greater good by providing health care to larger, broader segments of the general population. What theoretical framework is being used by this organization?

   a. deontologic theory
   b. virtue theory
   c. care theory
   d. teleologic theory

4. A nurse is working with a family who has recently learned their child has a terminal disease. The parents accept this after a time and are working with the grandparents to also accept the proposed outcome. When the grandparents ask the nurse if there is a good chance their grandchild will fully recover, the nurse replies, "No, your grandchild has a terminal illness and is not expected to live. I am very sorry for your family." The nurse is using which principle of ethics?

   a. fidelity
   b. justice
   c. veracity
   d. duty

5. A nurse offering a family a day pass to take the child out of the hospital to go to a movie theater for the afternoon is applying which of the following ethics principles?

    a. autonomy

    b. beneficence

    c. nonmaleficence

    d. privacy

6. Negligence by the nurse may be judged when the nurse:

    a. fails to meet the nurse's legal standard of care

    b. delegates to others appropriately

    c. makes an error in treatment that results in no harm to the client

    d. acts in good faith

7. In most states, an adult is defined as:

    a. any person legally married

    b. any person over the age of 16

    c. any person who pays taxes

    d. any person working part time

Multiple Response

1. Which of the following statements about the Health Insurance Portability and Accountability Act (HIPAA) are true? Select all that apply.

    a. HIPAA applies only to personal health information that is in the written format.

    b. HIPAA does not override mandatory reporting laws or state privacy laws that create a higher standard than the federal law.

    c. If an adolescent is seen at a clinic for confidential reproductive care, the parent cannot obtain the child's medical records unless written permission is given by the client.

    d. Client information should not be given over the phone unless the nurse is able to verify that the person receiving the information is someone entitled to that information under HIPAA regulations.

    e. HIPAA regulations become effective when the client turns 21 years of age.

    f. A client's HIPAA form must be renewed every year.

2. When providing teaching for a patient regarding a procedure, the nurse will include which of the following to address needed areas of informed consent? Select all that apply.

    a. risks of the procedure
    b. cost of the procedure
    c. alternatives to the procedure
    d. benefits of the procedure
    e. discharge instructions
    f. hazards of the procedure

3. Some of the following are recognized exceptions when a provider can breach client confidentiality. Select all that apply.

    a. infectious disease that needs to be reported to the local health department
    b. possibility of danger to a third party
    c. suspected abuse
    d. request of neighbors to be aware of potential health problem
    e. request of the grandparent of the client who is a minor
    f. request of the superintendent of a school district

4. In which of the following circumstances is confidentiality maintained? Select all that apply.

    a. sharing information with others for the purpose of developing a plan of care
    b. obtaining information for a friend of the family who is concerned
    c. updating other health care professionals involved in the care of the client
    d. gathering information to be used in utilization review for the health care facility
    e. providing information requested by a local news agency
    f. answering concerns for the parents of a married 18-year-old female

Critical Thinking/Case Study

An 8-year-old boy is brought to the emergency department by his caregiver. The caregiver reports the following: "Rajesh is just sleeping all of the time. He usually is very active. I think there is something wrong with him. I called his mother and she said he will be okay and that I should not keep calling her. I don't know how to contact his father; I don't know who his father is. I don't want to get in trouble, but I really think there is something wrong." Rajesh then starts to have a seizure while the nurse is completing the intake assessment.

1. Do members of the health care team need to call the family to obtain consent before treating Rajesh at this time?

   _____

   _____

   _____

2. Is it likely the caregiver will be sued by Rajesh's mother for slander?

   _____

   _____

   _____

3. Upon further assessment of Rajesh, the nurse suspects he is a victim of abuse based on lumps on his head, bruising inconsistent with common falls for an 8-year-old, and evidence of burns on his body. Does the mother need to consent to further evaluation of these injuries?

   _____

   _____

   _____

CHAPTER 3

The Child in Context of the Family

True or False

1. A genogram is a format for drawing a family tree that records information about family members and their relationships over a period of time, usually three generations.

   ❑ True   ❑ False

2. An in-depth family assessment should ideally include all family members and take place on neutral territory, such as a health care facility office.

   ❑ True   ❑ False

3. Children of gay and lesbian parents, compared to children of heterosexual parents, are more likely to be lesbian or gay.

   ❑ True   ❑ False

4. To provide culturally sensitive care to children and their families, the nurse must first be aware of his or her own values and beliefs and recognize how they influence his or her attitudes and actions.

   ❑ True   ❑ False

5. The United States has one of the lowest adolescent pregnancy rates among developed countries.

   ❑ True   ❑ False

6. Corporal punishment involves the application of some form of physical pain in response to undesired behavior.

   ❑ True   ❑ False

7. Susan is 14. She has a 1-month-old son who is experiencing health problems. Susan's parents are considered the decision makers for care of the baby.

   ❑ True   ❑ False

8. Parents of adopted children are now advised to openly discuss adoption from the beginning of their relationship with their child.

   ❑ True   ❑ False

9. Fathers in intact families today spend more time with their children than at any other time period in the past 100 years.

   ❑ True   ❑ False

10. The fundamental problem with the ABC-X model is that it is linear. It attempts to explain the complexity of family life and situations, though these events do not occur in a linear fashion. The accumulation of normative and nonnormative events over time often causes families to be stressed, and thus in crisis.

    ❑ True   ❑ False

Fill in the Blank

1. The _____ remains the basic social unit of society.

2. In the nursing theory by _____, the major goal of the nurse is to help keep the structure of the family stable within its environment.

3. In the nursing theory by _____, the goal of nursing is to promote adaptation and minimize ineffective responses.

4. The five functions that have been identified as important for nurses to understand in working with families are _____, _____, _____, _____, and _____.

5. _____ is general knowledge that is applied in family assessment and is initiated for identification and mitigation of risk factors associated with environmental stressors to prevent possible reaction.

6. _____ means having an awareness and appreciation of an influence in health care and being respectful of differences in cultural belief systems and values.

7. The _____ family consists of those members of the nuclear family and other blood-related persons such as grandparents, aunts, uncles, and cousins.

8. A _____ or _____ occurs when a divorced, widowed, or never-married single parent forms a household with a new partner who may or may not have a child or children.

Matching

_____ 1. Talmud

a. client is an individual, family, group, or community in constant interaction with a changing environment

_____ 2. Roy's Adaptation

b. giving to the poor theory

_____ 3. Ecomap

c. encyclopedia of commentaries on Jewish law

_____ 4. Zakat

d. family attributes and supports used in crisis situations

_____ 5. resources

e. visual representation of family in relation to community

Multiple Choice

1. Lafonda, age 8, is a recently diagnosed diabetic. She will require extensive teaching about diet, exercise, and medication administration to manage the disease process. Family members will need to be educated about this process. Which is the best question for the nurse to ask Lafonda about who the members of her family are?

   a. Does your father live at home with you?
   b. Who is your biologic mother?
   c. Who are the members of your family?
   d. Who are your parents and brothers and sisters?

2. Sophia, age 4, is starting the process of entering a stepfamily. Her parents have divorced. Sophia's father has remarried. Sophia's mother is single and living alone. Joint custody with equal time spent with the parents has been granted by the court. Based on her age, the nurse would expect Sophia to exhibit which one of the following as a transition to a stepfamily?

   a. acting out toward the stepparent in a negative way based on divided loyalties to the biologic parent
   b. magical thinking that she can reunite the divorced parents
   c. attempts to break up the new marriage
   d. development of psychosomatic symptoms

3. When providing information about parenting skills for a group of parents of adolescents, the nurse identifies the primary developmental-related parental task for adolescents as:

   a. supporting the child's growing autonomy in a safe environment
   b. promoting cognitive development
   c. helping the child to understand another's viewpoint
   d. maintaining open lines of communication

4. Which parenting style is characterized by the caregiver being warm but firm?

   a. authoritarian
   b. permissive
   c. indulgent
   d. indifferent

Multiple Response

1. In working with families, the nurse has chosen to use the Calgary Family Assessment Model. The nurse will gather information in which of the following major categories? Select all that apply.

   a. family structure
   b. family finance
   c. family development
   d. family functioning
   e. family educational level
   f. family health history

2. The nurse is teaching a group of preschool children healthy snacking habits. Kevin, age 4, is constantly acting up, not listening, and touching the other children. What actions are appropriate for the nurse? Select all that apply.

   a. Set clear rules about appropriate behavior before the talk begins.
   b. Explain the consequences to expect if the child does not follow the rules.
   c. Administer the consequences after the class so Kevin is not embarrassed in front of his friends.
   d. Praise Kevin when he is behaving appropriately.
   e. Use corporal punishment.
   f. Tell Kevin he will be removed from his preschool class unless he behaves.

3. Which of the following criteria should the nurse use when selecting a family assessment instrument? Select all that apply.

   a. language at the 11th grade level

   b. measures completed within 3 to 5 minutes

   c. measures that are sensitive to race

   d. measures that are sensitive to age

   e. measures that are sensitive to gender

   f. measures that are sensitive to ethnic background

Critical Thinking/Case Study

Casey is 7 years old. He was adopted by his parents and brought to the United States. Casey's parents ask the nurse some questions about the adoptive process. How could the nurse best respond to the following questions asked by the parents?

1. Our friends have an open adoption. We don't understand what that means. Can you tell us the difference between an open and closed adoption?

   _____

   _____

   _____

2. When do you think we should start to discuss with Casey the fact that he is adopted?

   _____

   _____

   _____

3. What can we do to ensure Casey grows up to be a happy and healthy person?

   _____

   _____

   _____

CHAPTER 4

Community and Home Health Nursing

True or False

1. The community health nurse has a focus on health promotion and disease prevention.

   ❑ True ❑ False

2. Medicare covers optional services determined by individual states such as dental care; speech, hearing, and language disorders; and eyeglasses.

   ❑ True ❑ False

3. All states have an Early and Periodic Screening Diagnosis and Treatment Program (EPSDT) that offers early screening, diagnosis, treatment, and periodic follow-up services to children and youth under 21 years of age who meet the financial eligibility requirements.

   ❑ True ❑ False

4. Managed care refers to a cost-effective delivery of health care services.

   ❑ True ❑ False

5. Children who are technology-dependent and those who need hospice care receive the majority of home care nursing hours.

   ❑ True ❑ False

6. When referring to interpersonal relationships, the nurse-client relationship should occur in the zone closest to distancing/disinterested to be helpful.

   ❑ True ❑ False

7. Relief care is short-term, temporary care and provides relief to families that care for a child who requires specialized care.

   ❑ True ❑ False

8. A windshield survey is a systematic assessment that is performed while the nurse travels through the community.

   ❑ True ❑ False

9. The effects of lead on the central nervous system are reversible.

   ❏ True   ❏ False

10. It is expected that the need for home health care nursing for children and their families will continue to grow in the future.

    ❏ True   ❏ False

Fill in the Blank

1. Various roles of the community health nurse include _____, _____, _____, _____, _____, _____, _____, and _____.

2. _____ is defined as activities or interventions that identify risk factors related to disease, the lifestyle changes related to disease prevention, and the process of enabling individuals and communities to increase control over and improve their health. These activities or strategies are directed toward developing the resources of clients to maintain or enhance their physical, social, emotional, and spiritual well-being.

3. _____ is defined as activities designed to maintain the current level of health, actively prevent disease, detect disease early, and thwart disease processes or maintain functioning within constraints of the disease.

4. _____ refers to those activities designed to protect persons from disease and its consequences.

5. _____ is directed toward children with clinically apparent disease.

6. _____ is short-term, temporary care that is normally provided in the home for a child who requires specialized care; it provides relief for the caregivers, which may help to prevent burnout and increase the caregivers' ability to cope with the stress.

Matching

_____ 1. case manager

_____ 2. counselor

a. speaks for the needs of a family that is facing homelessness with a child who is dependent on technology

b. works with caregivers to decide if their child, who is dependent on technology, should attend school or be tutored at home

_____ 3. researcher

c. identifies an area where environmental toxins near a popular playground are jeopardizing the health of children, and develops solutions that will promote health and well-being

_____ 4. advocate

d. coordinates all the services (occupational therapy, physical therapy, tutoring, as well as financial resources for the caregiver) needed by a child recuperating from a hospital stay to ensure a healthy recovery

Multiple Choice

1. The community health nurse working in a given area with people concerned about environmental toxins should perform which of the following activities first?

   a. Teach the families to minimize household chemicals.
   b. Screen basements for radon.
   c. Obtain serum lead levels of children in the area.
   d. Assess the site environment.

2. Which of the following is not an example of health promotion activities?

   a. well-child care clinics
   b. nutrition programs
   c. immunization clinics
   d. sanitation measures

3. When teaching primary preventative strategies about lead poisoning, the nurse would include which one of the following statements?

   a. "A diet high in protein will reverse any lead levels your child may have."
   b. "Adequate calcium intake will reduce the absorption of lead."
   c. "A diet high in carbohydrates will increase lead levels in the blood."
   d. "High-fiber foods will reduce the absorption of lead."

4. To establish professional boundaries when working with families in the home, the nurse will:

    a. make families aware of their vulnerability
    b. inform the family that the nurse is there to meet all of their needs
    c. use themselves as an example of how to live a healthy lifestyle
    d. include caregivers into the plan of care

5. The home care nurse has been assigned to work with a newborn who is receiving photo-therapy and antibiotic therapy. The nurse meets the newborn and family and performs an assessment. Which phase of the home visit is the nurse in?

    a. preinteraction
    b. engagement
    c. active
    d. termination

Multiple Response

1. Components of a community assessment by a community health nurse include which of the following? Select all that apply.

    a. What is the child's neighborhood like?
    b. Which diseases are most common in the community?
    c. What is the availability and funding of health care resources?
    d. Are there adequate community resources available?
    e. What do most residents die from?
    f. How many individuals living in the area receive public assistance?

2. Which statements does the nurse include when teaching a group of caregivers about the effects of lead poisoning? Select all that apply.

    a. Lead poisoning has the most effect on the renal system.
    b. Lead is removed from the body by chelation therapy.
    c. Acute encephalopathy is a manifestation of lead poisoning.
    d. Hypertension can be a manifestation of lead poisoning.
    e. Lead poisoning is not a concern in the new millennium.
    f. The only type of lead that is problematic is lead that is used in paint in the inside of houses.

3. In the role of case manager when working with a 10-year-old ventilator-dependent child, the nurse has which responsibilities? Select all that apply.

   a. coordination of all care the child receives

   b. assessment of the availability of community resources needed by the family

   c. management of the family's financial situation to be able to meet health care costs

   d. evaluation of the effectiveness of the coordination of care for the family

   e. implementation of a fund-raising program to support the family and child

   f. certification of the need for assistance programs

Critical Thinking/Case Study

The home health nurse has been assigned to care for a Bosnian family who has recently entered the United States. The 7-year-old son is recovering from heart surgery for repair of a ventricular septal defect.

1. Who controls the setting for care in the home?

   _____

   _____

   _____

2. How should the nurse respond to a home that is cluttered and in disarray?

   _____

   _____

   _____

3. Give examples of how the nurse can determine family roles and tasks among all members.

   _____

   _____

   _____

CHAPTER 5

School Nursing

True or False

1. School nursing owes its beginnings in both the United States and Europe to the field of medical-surgical nursing.

   ❑ True ❑ False

2. Because of the passage of federal laws such as the Individuals with Disabilities Education Act, these children have the right to an educational experience, provided in their home, that is similar to that of every other child in the United States.

   ❑ True ❑ False

3. The role of the school nurse in screening programs is to refer children for further evaluation, and correction if necessary, when abnormalities are noted.

   ❑ True ❑ False

4. Many teens feel nothing bad can happen to them; it only happens to other people.

   ❑ True ❑ False

5. Due to media attention describing the negative health risks of tobacco, the number of people who smoke cigarettes has significantly decreased over the last several years.

   ❑ True ❑ False

6. Because children do not complain when they have vision or hearing problems, it may be overlooked.

   ❑ True ❑ False

7. Automatic external defibrillator (AED) machines may only be used on individuals 18 years of age or older.

   ❑ True ❑ False

8. Most school districts still require caregiver and physician permission for the use of herbal therapies at school even if they can be purchased over the counter.

   ❑ True ❑ False

9. Bullying has been shown to leave long-term psychological effects, such as insecurity, loneliness, and depression.

   ❑ True ❑ False

10. When working with children, the school nurse must follow federal and state HIPAA regulations.

    ❑ True ❑ False

Fill in the Blank

1. The school nurse is involved in many school health services. _____ includes providing nursing procedures or care to individual students; _____ includes consulting with staff on behalf of a child's health needs and providing community referrals and health education.

2. The school nurse's role in communicable disease control revolves around the three factors necessary for spread: _____, _____, and _____.

3. _____ has been shown to be an effective way to decrease the spread of communicable disease from the direct contact route.

4. Diseases that can spread quickly through the classroom and lead to complications in some children include _____, _____, and _____.

5. Children who are overweight are at a higher risk for the development of _____, _____, and _____, which puts them at risk for chronic health problems as adults.

6. A(n) _____ is a document, based on a nurse's assessment of a child, that outlines the special health needs, goals, interventions, and outcomes necessary to improve or maintain the health of the child and allow him or her to remain in school.

7. The process of getting high using aerosol products such as cleaners, solvents, adhesives, hair spray, or even whipped cream is called _____ or _____.

8. The school nurse's main focus in child abuse or neglect issues is _____.

Matching

_____ 1. phoria   a. excessive farsightedness

_____ 2. strabismus   b. permanent vision loss

_____ 3. scoliosis   c. muscle balance of the eye

_____ 4. hyperopia   d. lazy eye

_____ 5. amblyopia   e. lateral curvature of the spine

Multiple Choice

1. Referral for further evaluation should occur when the school-age child does not have visual acuity of:

   a. 20/10

   b. 20/20

   c. 20/30

   d. 20/40

2. Scoliosis is most often seen in which age group?

   a. 3-year-olds

   b. 8-year-olds

   c. 12-year-olds

   d. 17-year-olds

3. When working with caregivers of a child diagnosed with mild attention-deficit disorder (ADD) or attention-deficit hyperactivity disorder (ADHD), the school nurse informs the caregivers that:

   a. The child will be placed in a special classroom for children with this disorder.

   b. Along with medication as prescribed, other measures used in working with the child include behavior modification, counseling, and classroom interventions.

   c. Ritalin, a drug commonly used in the treatment of ADD/ADHD, is a depressant used to suppress overactivity.

   d. Their child will carry the medication with them and take it as needed.

4. A school nurse is working with an assistant who is not licensed. There are several children in the nurse's office who are in need of some form of attention. The nurse may delegate all but which one of the following tasks to the assistant?

   a. obtaining a blood sugar level on a child who has an insulin pump for the treatment of diabetes mellitus

   b. irrigation of a colostomy

   c. assessment of a patient's response to treatment for hypoglycemia

   d. bandaging of a scraped knee

Multiple Response

1. Which of the following are preventative procedures performed by the school nurse? Select all that apply.

   a. first aid for a cut obtained on the playground

   b. curriculum development on drug and violence prevention

   c. vision and hearing screenings

   d. education in nutrition

   e. review of immunization history for the child

   f. treatment for lice

2. Which of the following regulations for medication administration will the school nurse follow? Select all that apply.

   a. All medications must be stored in a locked cabinet.

   b. All medications must be labeled by a pharmacist.

   c. Unlicensed personnel may be assigned to administer the medication.

   d. The school must have written orders from the physician for administration of the medication.

   e. The school nurse must have written permission from the child's caregiver for administration of the medication.

   f. Follow the local health care facility's policies and procedures in medication administration as these cover the school.

3. The school nurse expects to find which of the following upon assessment of a school-age child who uses stimulants? Select all that apply.

   a. constricted pupils

   b. restlessness

   c. increased body temperature

   d. euphoria

   e. tremors

   f. ptosis

4. Which of the following are components of an Individual Health Plan (IHP) for a child in school? Select all that apply.

   a. baseline assessment data

   b. nutritional considerations

   c. an emergency plan individualized for each child

   d. daily cost of caring for the child incurred by the school district

   e. medications taken by the child at home and at school

   f. daily cost of caring for the child incurred by the family

5. A school nurse is responsible for the care of a child who has a "Do Not Attempt to Resuscitate" (DNAR) order at school. The nurse will do which of the following? Select all that apply.

   a. Refuse to care for this child in the school setting.

   b. Notify local emergency management providers and set up a plan so that if the child has an event at school, palliative care will be rendered.

   c. Ensure that the DNAR order is dated within a monthly time frame.

   d. Educate the staff that a DNAR order can be revoked verbally by a parent at any time.

   e. Inform the staff that in some states, resuscitating a person with a written DNAR order present is considered assault and battery and is punishable by law.

   f. Perform CPR if needed because it is the nurse's responsibility to save all children.

6. Which of the following does the school nurse identify as symptoms of a child who is being bullied? Select all that apply.

   a. frequent psychosomatic complaints

   b. school avoidance

   c. sleeplessness

   d. depression

   e. attempted suicide

   f. improvement in school performance

Critical Thinking/Case Study

Maria is 9 years old. She has transferred to the school from another state. Upon checking the admission forms, the school nurse notes that Maria has received none of the state-mandated immunizations for entry into school. The nurse informs the caregivers that Maria needs to be up-to-date with all immunizations before entry into school. The caregivers have several questions for the nurse. How could the nurse best respond to the following questions asked by the caregivers?

1. I don't understand; she did not have these shots at the other school. Why do you say she has to have them?

   _____

   _____

   _____

2. We don't even have a family doctor yet. How do you expect us to take care of all of this?

   _____

   _____

   _____

3. I've heard that a lot of times kids get really sick after they get those immunization shots. Why should I risk my child getting sick from the shots?

   _____

   _____

   _____

CHAPTER 6

Theoretical Approaches to the Growth and Development of Children

True or False

1. In toddlerhood, the characteristic of human development is forming attachments to family and other caregivers.

   ❑ True   ❑ False

2. Cephalocaudal development proceeds from the head downward.

   ❑ True   ❑ False

3. Development follows a set pattern for every child.

   ❑ True   ❑ False

4. Caregivers should be reminded of the importance of recognizing that physiologic, psychosocial, and cognitive development are separate developmental entities.

   ❑ True   ❑ False

5. Erikson acknowledged the contribution of biologic factors to development but felt that the environment, culture, and society are also important.

   ❑ True   ❑ False

6. The third developmental stage by Erikson, covering 3 to 6 years of age, is autonomy versus shame and doubt.

   ❑ True   ❑ False

7. Sullivan focused on interpersonal relations as important behavioral motivators and the source of psychological health.

   ❑ True   ❑ False

8. The behavioral perspective posits that human actions and interactions come from learned responses to environmental stimuli.

   ❑ True   ❑ False

9. Although gender stereotyping is declining, it still occurs and can affect a child's development, especially if he or she is treated according to rigid role characteristics.

   ❑ True   ❑ False

10. Ecological theory helps us understand that human development can proceed along several different pathways, depending on the interplay of internal and external forces within the individual.

    ❑ True   ❑ False

Fill in the Blank

1. _____ describes genetically inherited traits such as eye color and body type, and diseases such as hemophilia.

2. _____ suggests change is orderly and built upon earlier experiences.

3. The _____ refers to a limited time span when a child is biologically prepared to acquire certain behaviors.

4. Freud originated the _____ theory, emphasizing the importance of unconscious motivation and early childhood experiences in influencing behavior, and describing concepts related to personality and early childhood stages of development.

5. To Freud, the most important life instinct is the _____ instinct, which changes its character and focus according to biologic maturation.

6. _____ assumed humans are rational creatures whose actions, feelings, and thoughts are controlled primarily by the ego instead of the id, superego, or conflicts among the three components of the personality.

7. The period of infancy was described by Freud as _____, while Erikson called this period _____ and Piaget referred to it as _____.

8. The two most important points stressed by Sullivan are (1) the significance of _____ with others on personality development and (2) meeting the child's _____ in a timely and appropriate fashion.

9. To Piaget, interactions with the environment cause people to organize patterns of thought or _____, which they use to interpret or make sense of their experiences.

10. Sidman developed several criteria to evaluate how useful a theory is, including _____, _____, _____, _____, _____, and _____.

Matching

_____ 1. social learning

_____ 2. id

_____ 3. Kohlberg

_____ 4. latency

_____ 5. tabula rasa

_____ 6. ecology (Bronfenbrenner)

_____ 7. original sin

_____ 8. maturation

_____ 9. superego

_____ 10. Bandura

_____ 11. Electra complex

_____ 12. adolescence

a. all psychic energy

b. changes due to genetic inheritance rather than life experience, illness, or injury

c. contextual perspective

d. children learn by imitating and observing others (model)

e. fascination with gender differences

f. children are inherently evil and selfish egotists who must be controlled by society

g. conscience

h. operational thought begins

i. behavioral perspective

j. formulated a theory of moral development

k. appropriate gender roles adopted

l. children are born neither good nor evil and are molded through life experiences

Multiple Choice

1. When working with families, the nurse chooses to use the behavioral perspective. The nurse would most likely follow a theory developed by:

   a. Skinner

   b. Erikson

   c. Piaget

   d. Bronfenbrenner

2. When explaining Freudian theory to a group of caregivers, the nurse states that according to this theory, two basic biologic instincts motivate behavior, must be satisfied, and compete for supremacy. They are:

   a. sleep and play

   b. hunger and food

   c. feeling loved and being touched

   d. life and death

3. According to Freud's stages of psychosexual development, a 12-year-old would be in which stage?

   a. anal

   b. phallic

   c. latency

   d. genital

4. A nurse working with a 10-year-old is following Erikson's psychosocial theory of development. The nurse correctly identifies the child as being in which stage of development?

   a. autonomy versus shame and doubt

   b. initiative versus guilt

   c. industry versus inferiority

   d. identity versus role confusion

5. According to Sullivan's interpersonal theory of development, the importance of "chum" relationships occurs at which stage?

   a. late childhood

   b. preadolescence

   c. early adolescence

   d. late adolescence

6. Social learning, a kind of behaviorism, was proposed by:

   a. Bandura

   b. Skinner

   c. Freud

   d. Erikson

7. Application of ecological theory into care of the child incorporates which one of the following?

   a. The child's world is composed of two important systems, internal and external.
   b. The child is viewed as separate parts of physical and emotional components.
   c. Stress or illness in one family member will affect the entire family system.
   d. All children in the family go through the same family experience.

Multiple Response

1. When teaching a parenting class, the nurse chooses to apply Freudian theory to provide insight into human actions. The nurse will incorporate which of the following statements? Select all that apply.

   a. During infancy, comfort and pleasure are obtained through the mouth.
   b. Toddlers are gratified by controlling body excretions.
   c. Preschool children are most concerned about controlling their environment.
   d. School-age children should be encouraged to have contact with friends.
   e. Adolescents vacillate between dependence and independence from parents.
   f. Any attraction toward the parent of the opposite sex is considered to be a reason for concern.

2. Application of Erikson's developmental theory in the care of children includes which of the following? Select all that apply.

   a. assessing the five developmental crises children and adolescents face
   b. maintaining variety in daily routines for toddlers to prevent boredom
   c. providing opportunities for continuing schoolwork if the school-age child is hospitalized
   d. encouraging adolescents to take responsibility for their own actions
   e. accepting a child's choice and negative expression of feelings
   f. determining menu choices for all hospitalized children to ensure adequate nutritional intake

3. The nurse is asked to summarize the theories of Skinner and operant conditioning. The nurse will include which of the following statements? Select all that apply.

    a. Behavioral change becomes more permanent when consequences are provided continuously rather than intermittently.

    b. Skinner emphasized why behaviors occur rather than simply describing the behaviors.

    c. Operant conditioning involves behavioral change due to either negative or positive consequences rather than just the occurrence of a stimulus.

    d. Punishment includes a frown or withdrawal of privileges.

    e. The child must successfully achieve in one developmental level to progress to the next.

    f. Infants' needs are met by oral satisfaction.

Critical Thinking

Compare and contrast theories of human development proposed by Bandura, Freud, Piaget, and Bronfenbrenner.

_____

_____

_____

CHAPTER 7

Growth and Development of the Newborn

True or False

1. A positive Babinski's reflex in an 18-month-old is indicative of cerebral palsy.

   ❏ True   ❏ False

2. In the newborn, mediastinal structures in conjunction with a relatively large heart reduce the space available for lung expansion.

   ❏ True   ❏ False

3. The liver of the newborn remains functionally immature until approximately 6 months of age.

   ❏ True   ❏ False

4. Blood on the diaper of the newborn female is due to the withdrawal of maternal hormones at the time of delivery and is considered normal.

   ❏ True   ❏ False

5. Habituation protects the newborn from overstimulation and frees energy to meet physiologic demands.

   ❏ True   ❏ False

6. All newborns receive ophthalmic drops or ointment shortly after birth to prevent the transfer of syphilis from the mother to the infant at the time of delivery.

   ❏ True   ❏ False

7. In recent studies, the back sleeping position has been shown to produce a large and sustained decrease in the incidence of sudden infant death syndrome (SIDS).

   ❏ True   ❏ False

8. The increase in neonatal morbidity and mortality in the postmature infant is most likely due to pulmonary insufficiency.

   ❏ True   ❏ False

Fill in the Blank

1. The neonatal or newborn period is defined as the first _____ of life.

2. Fetal circulation is different from neonatal circulation due to structural differences that include _____, _____, _____, _____, and _____.

3. The swelling of the soft tissues of the scalp in the newborn is called _____. A collection of blood between the skull bone and the periosteum as a result of the rupture of blood vessels secondary to head trauma from birth is called _____.

4. The posterior fontanel typically closes by _____ months of age, while the anterior fontanel closes between _____ months of age.

5. In the newborn, the heart rate will range from _____ beats per minute while asleep to _____ beats per minute while awake.

6. _____ is a form of newborn jaundice in which nuclear masses of the brain and spinal cord undergo pathologic changes accompanied by the deposition of bile pigments within them. It can occur when levels of bilirubin reach toxic levels.

7. The primary form of heat production in the newborn is through metabolism of _____.

8. _____, or the use of special high-intensity fluorescent lights, is generally an effective method of reducing serum bilirubin levels and preventing kernicterus.

9. In the newborn, _____ are small white papules on the nose, face, forehead, and upper torso caused by the plugging of sebaceous glands; _____ are small, pinpoint, nonraised, perfectly round, purplish-red spots that are a result of an intradermal or submucosal hemorrhage; and a _____ is an irregularly dark pigmented area on the posterior lumbar region.

10. _____ is a congenital defect in the walls of the spinal cord caused by a lack of union between the laminae of the vertebrae.

11. Another name for clubfoot is _____.

12. The newborn is more vulnerable to underheating and overheating because of _____, _____, _____, and _____.

13. Bedding that has been associated with a higher incidence of sudden infant death syndrome (SIDS) includes such items as _____, _____, _____, and _____.

Matching

_____ 1. kernicterus

_____ 2. hydrocele

_____ 3. foramen ovale

_____ 4. desquamation

_____ 5. caput succedaneum

a. opening between the right and left atria

b. swelling of the soft tissue of the scalp which may extend across the suture lines

c. chronic and permanent sequelae of bilirubin toxicity

d. collection of fluid between the parietal and visceral layers of the tunica vaginalis

e. peeling of the skin

Multiple Choice

1. Janet, a nurse working in the newborn nursery, is providing care to Abe, a newborn in need of phototherapy. Which one of the following interventions will Janet perform in Abe's care?

   a. assessment for dehydration and excoriation of the skin in the perianal area due to loose stools and increased urine output

   b. repositioning of Abe once a shift

   c. application of ophthalmic ointment every two hours to protect Abe's eyes

   d. positioning the light source to shine on Abe's liver while shielding the rest of his body

2. Janiqua asks the nurse, "How should I take care of my son's circumcision? It looks so painful; I don't want to hurt him." The best response by the nurse would be:

   a. Any yellow color around the circumcised area is considered a sign of infection. Call the primary care provider immediately should you notice this.

   b. Apply a thick layer of an antibiotic cream to the area three times daily to prevent infection.

   c. Any tissue you see forming around the circumcised area should not be removed.

   d. Change diapers infrequently to avoid trauma to the circumcised area.

3. Marilyn asks the nurse, "I don't want my new baby Tracy to get diaper rash. How do babies get this rash?" Which statement would the nurse omit from her response?

   a. Diaper rash can be caused by an allergic reaction to diaper material.

   b. It can be caused by too much moisture next to the skin.

   c. Diaper rash can be caused by the baby's skin rubbing against the diaper.

   d. Diaper rash is caused by bacterial contamination. It is passed from baby to baby when the caregiver does not properly wash his or her hands between the care of each baby.

4. When teaching families how to maintain body temperature of the newborn, which statement made by the new nurse requires the supervising nurse to intervene?

   a. Block sunlight on the newborn in the car to prevent overheating.

   b. Place the newborn's crib next to the window.

   c. Warm solid surfaces beneath the newborn by placing a blanket on the surface.

   d. Reduce areas of the skin exposed during a bath.

5. Which of the following actions by a mother learning how to breastfeed her infant requires the nurse to intervene? The mother:

   a. burps the baby after feeding from each breast

   b. burps the baby at the end of the feeding

   c. cleanses her nipples with alcohol before breastfeeding the baby

   d. places the baby's lips so they encircle the areola when breastfeeding

6. An infant who is large for gestational age would not be at increased risk for a:

   a. broken clavicle

   b. fractured humerus

   c. caput succedaneum

   d. hyperglycemia

7. Which of the following is not a symptom of respiratory distress syndrome in the newborn?

   a. respiratory rate of 40 breaths per minute

   b. sternal retractions

   c. nasal flaring

   d. audible grunting

Multiple Response

1. Jennifer has just given birth to her first child. She has many questions and concerns about the care of her newborn son, and asks the nurse, "How am I supposed to take care of his belly button? It looks really sore." Which of the following statements by the nurse are appropriate? Select all that apply.

   a. Be sure to keep the umbilical cord covered by the diaper.
   b. Use 70% isopropyl alcohol or hydrogen peroxide to cleanse the umbilical cord while attached.
   c. Continue to use the 70% isopropyl alcohol or hydrogen peroxide to the cord area after the cord falls off until the skin appears normal.
   d. Do not attempt to loosen the cord or pull it off.
   e. The cord should stay attached for four weeks to prevent infection.
   f. The baby will not feel any pain when you clean around it.

2. Which of the following are acceptable variances found in a newborn physical assessment? Select all that apply.

   a. eyelid edema
   b. resting heart rate of 80
   c. supernumerary nipples
   d. functional heart murmur
   e. hands reach knees when arms extended to the side
   f. cephalhematoma

3. Britt, mother of 1-day-old Crystal, tells the nurse, "I know some people put their babies on formula, but I just can't afford it. There is no way I am going to nurse my baby. I am giving Crystal regular milk that I drink as soon as I get out of here." How should the nurse respond? Select all that apply.

   a. Cow's milk differs significantly from human milk or commercial formulas.
   b. Cow's milk is not easily digested by babies.
   c. Cow's milk should be used for those infants allergic to formula.
   d. Cow's milk contains more fat and other substances than human milk or formula.
   e. You have the right to do what you think is best for your baby.
   f. I am going to have to contact children's services now that I know this is your plan.

Critical Thinking/Case Study

Mercedes is a student nurse. Her clinical instructor has asked Mercedes to give a presentation to her clinical group on the general appearance of the newborn. Help Mercedes prepare for her talk by answering the following questions.

1. What can Mercedes tell the group regarding the appearance of the newborn's head? What are some of the normal variations that can be expected?

   _____

   _____

   _____

2. What information should Mercedes include concerning fontanels?

   _____

   _____

   _____

3. How should Mercedes describe the typical appearance of the newborn's eyes and eyelids?

   _____

   _____

   _____

4. Skin color of the newborn should be addressed by Mercedes. What do you suggest she mention?

   _____

   _____

   _____

5. What information should Mercedes share with her clinical group regarding the appearance of the newborn's abdomen?

   _____

   _____

   _____

6. What types of visual aids could Mercedes use to enhance learning for members of her clinical group?

_____

_____

_____

CHAPTER 8

Growth and Development of the Infant

True or False

1. The age range for an infant is defined as 1 day to 2 years of age.

   ❑ True   ❑ False

2. By the end of the first year of life, the infant's birth weight will have doubled.

   ❑ True   ❑ False

3. By the end of two months, the primitive grasp reflex fades and the infant begins to actively grasp and momentarily hold an object before dropping it.

   ❑ True   ❑ False

4. Health screenings for the infant begin at the first visit to the primary care provider's office after birth.

   ❑ True   ❑ False

5. By approximately 8 to 12 months of age, an infant can recognize familiar faces and stranger anxiety may appear.

   ❑ True   ❑ False

6. Failure to turn toward a sound by 6 months of age is a behavior that should alert the nurse to an infant's possible hearing problems.

   ❑ True   ❑ False

7. Aspirin is the recommended medication for infants who are experiencing discomfort from teething.

   ❑ True   ❑ False

8. Finger foods for the older infant should be cut into the size of the caregiver's thumb.

   ❑ True   ❑ False

9. If the infant is weaned too soon from breast milk or formula, iron deficiency anemia could occur.

   ❏ True   ❏ False

10. Some characteristics of an infant with a difficult personality type include the need for a structured environment and slow adaptation to stimuli.

    ❏ True   ❏ False

11. According to Piaget, the major task of infancy is object permanence, in which the infant learns that an object is not an extension of self and that it continues to exist even when it cannot be seen.

    ❏ True   ❏ False

12. For infants under 2 months of age, it is recommended that a health care provider be made aware of a fever above 30.0°C (100.4°F).

    ❏ True   ❏ False

Fill in the Blank

1. As the head of the infant grows, the fontanels gradually close, with the posterior fontanel closing by _____ and the anterior fontanel closing by _____.

2. Gross motor development of the infant is assessed by the infant's ability to use large muscle groups to _____, _____, and _____.

3. By _____ months of age, the infant can hold an object securely and bang the hands together.

4. In the first year of life, health screenings are usually scheduled when the infant is 2 weeks old, and _____, _____, _____, _____, and 12 months old.

5. After an infant receives an MMR immunization, the caregiver may expect the infant to have a mild rash, low-grade fever, and drowsiness beginning _____ to _____ days after immunization.

6. The first teeth to erupt are referred to as the _____, _____, or _____ teeth.

7. By 12 months of age, the infant should have _____ teeth.

8. Usually the first food introduced to the infant is _____, since it is easy to digest and unlikely to cause allergy.

9. _____ is the most common food allergy encountered in the first year of life.

10. _____, one of the most common health problems seen in infants younger than 3 months of age, describes recurrent episodes of unexplained crying and inability to be consoled.

Matching

_____ 1. temperament

_____ 2. weaning

_____ 3. cruising

_____ 4. colic

_____ 5. seborrhea

a. cradle cap

b. deliberate steps while holding onto something

c. the way the child interacts with the surrounding environment

d. infant irritability

e. the process of giving up one method of feeding for another

Multiple Choice

1. A nurse is performing an assessment to determine gross motor development of a 4-month-old infant. The nurse expects to observe which of the following as age-appropriate development for this infant?

   a. head control demonstrated as ability to turn head from side to side, but inability to lift the head

   b. ability to hold head up and use forearms for support

   c. ability to hold head, chest, and abdomen up by bearing weight on the hands

   d. ability to sit alone without support

2. Marcella, a first-time mother, asks the nurse when she can expect her daughter Seneca, age 2 months, to start to crawl. The best response by the nurse is:

   a. 4 months

   b. 6 months

   c. 8 months

   d. 10 months

3. When teaching caregivers about visual development of the infant, the nurse includes which of the following?

   a. Infants are unable to see at the time of birth because the nerves for vision are immature.

   b. By 2 months of age, the infant can recognize familiar faces and stranger anxiety may appear.

   c. Infants prefer to look at pastel colors.

   d. Absent or poor hand-eye coordination by 7 months of age is a possible behavior related to visual problems.

4. A nurse is asked to teach a group of new parents infant dental care. Which one of the following statements will the nurse include in the talk?

   a. The teething process typically begins around 9 months of age.

   b. The first teeth to erupt are usually the back side teeth.

   c. Infants should not receive fluoridated water until after the first year of life.

   d. Schedule the first dental visit when the child is 2 years of age.

5. Rita is a 16-year-old who has a 1-month-old son named Kyle. Rita is overwhelmed by the care of her infant son. She asks the nurse, "When can I start to give Kyle food to feed himself?" The nurse responds that the time frame when most infants are ready for finger food is between:

   a. 2 and 4 months of age

   b. 4 and 6 months of age

   c. 6 and 8 months of age

   d. 8 and 10 months of age

6. A mother is planning to use a pacifier for her newborn. Which statement by the mother indicates more teaching about pacifier safety is needed?

   a. I will never place the pacifier on a string.

   b. I will use a pacifier with two-piece construction.

   c. The mouth guard of the pacifier should be wider than the infant's mouth.

   d. Ventilation holes should be present on the mouth guard of the pacifier.

7. Katie, age 2 months, cries for more than three hours a day, and more than three times a week. The situation has been going on for five weeks. Katie's mom, Kim, is tired and upset. She asks the nurse, "What am I to do with her? The doctor told me she has colic. How will I ever manage caring for a baby that cries all the time?" The nurse includes which of the following when teaching Kim how to care for a baby with colic?

   a. Avoid car rides, as Katie will most likely become more irritable due to the vibration and movement.

   b. Place Katie in a side-lying position during feeding.

   c. Walk or rock Katie while applying gentle pressure to her abdomen.

   d. Keep Katie uncovered to prevent her from feeling swaddled in a blanket wrap.

8. Which statement by the mother of a newborn indicates more education regarding sleep and the infant is indicated?

   a. Infants should be woken during a sleep period if the caregiver suspects the diaper is in need of changing.

   b. A 2-month-old typically sleeps about 16 hours a day.

   c. Most infants sleep through the night at 3 to 4 months of age.

   d. Sleeping with an infant increases the chances of suffocation.

9. The nurse assesses which of the following infants as being most at risk for the development of sudden infant death syndrome (SIDS)?

   a. Jack who sleeps in the supine position

   b. Jason who is 6 months of age

   c. John who is exposed to cigarette smoke in his home

   d. Jeb who received his MMR vaccination that day

10. Meesha is the mother of Mariah who is 12 months old. Meesha has much guilt associated with Mariah's outbursts when she leaves her at the babysitter's to go to work. The best advice the nurse can give Meesha for dealing with Mariah's separation anxiety is:

   a. Do not leave Mariah at the babysitter's without saying goodbye to her.

   b. Encourage the babysitter to take Mariah from you, even if she cries, to avoid a prolonged unpleasant experience for everyone.

   c. Remove any items at the babysitter's that may remind Mariah of you so she will not think of you during the day.

   d. Ask the babysitter not to speak to Mariah until after you leave so Mariah will have as much time with you as possible.

11. The nurse is assessing the home environment of an 8-month-old infant for safety promotion and injury prevention. Which of the following is considered unsafe and a potential cause of injury?

    a. Hot water heater thermostat is set at less than 120 degrees.

    b. Cords for blinds are out of reach.

    c. Pots on the stove have handles facing the front of the stove.

    d. Spaces between bed rail slats are 2 inches.

Multiple Response

1. The nurse expects which of the following tests to be completed as part of routine screening for the newborn? Select all that apply.

    a. HIV status

    b. PKU

    c. thyroid function

    d. hematocrit

    e. hemoglobin

    f. lead level

2. Family teaching for the family of the infant who has received routine immunizations includes which of the following? Select all that apply.

    a. Most common reactions last five to seven days.

    b. Irritability is a common reaction to immunization.

    c. Redness at the injection site is common.

    d. Mild loss of appetite is expected.

    e. Swelling at the injection site is common.

    f. Tenderness at the injection site is common.

3. While performing an assessment on a 9-month-old infant, the nurse notes the following behaviors. Which may indicate that the infant has a hearing problem? Select all that apply.

    a. lack of startle or blink reflex with a loud sound

    b. cooing or babbling sounds by the infant

    c. failure to turn head toward sound by 6 months of age

    d. failure to follow verbal direction

    e. irritation with loud sounds

    f. preoccupation with sucking

4. At a routine office visit, the caregiver of a 5-month-old infant asks the nurse to explain about feeding the baby solid food. The nurse will include which of the following? Select all that apply.

   a. Introduce one new food every other day to allow for identifying food allergies.
   b. Feed solids with a spoon.
   c. Place food toward the back middle of the infant's mouth.
   d. Give solid foods when the infant is hungry, then follow with formula or breast milk.
   e. Introduce the infant to vegetables before fruits.
   f. Gradually increase solid food to approximately 8 ounces per day.

Critical Thinking/Case Study

The nurse is asked to provide information on normal growth and development, parenting techniques, and health promotion to a group of about twelve caregivers of eight infants ranging from 1 month to 14 months of age.

1. How can the nurse best explain physiological development of the infant in the first 12 months of life?

   _____

   _____

   _____

2. What can the caregivers expect to see as the infant develops fine and gross motor skills as well as locomotion?

   _____

   _____

   _____

3. Summarize for the caregivers health screenings performed on the newborn, when they will be performed in the first year of life, and parameters of when the health care provider should be called if illness is suspected in the infant.

   _____

   _____

   _____

4. Explain development of the visual and auditory systems of the infant.

   _____

   _____

   _____

5. Summarize infant feeding progression from milk to semisolid and solid food.

   _____

   _____

   _____

6. Describe the characteristics of a childproof home and assist caregivers in adapting their homes to meet these standards.

   _____

   _____

   _____

CHAPTER 9

Growth and Development of the Toddler

True or False

1. The average weight gain during toddlerhood is about two pounds per year.

   ❏ True ❏ False

2. Masturbation is common in toddlerhood and should be handled in a matter-of-fact manner, thereby lessening the child's anxiety and feelings of shame.

   ❏ True ❏ False

3. Erikson refers to the time of toddlerhood as trust versus mistrust.

   ❏ True ❏ False

4. Most parents in the United States use corporal punishment in disciplining their children.

   ❏ True ❏ False

5. Nurses should never physically discipline a child.

   ❏ True ❏ False

6. Consistent day and night dryness should be achieved by 3 years of age or further evaluation for physical or psychological problems is warranted.

   ❏ True ❏ False

7. Play has been described as "the work of childhood."

   ❏ True ❏ False

8. Most 2-year-olds require 10–12 hours of sleep each day.

   ❏ True ❏ False

9. The child's first visit to the dentist should be soon after the first teeth erupt at about 2 years of age.

   ❏ True ❏ False

10. To encourage a child to take medication, never tell the child that it is candy.

    ❑ True   ❑ False

11. The pot-bellied appearance of toddlers is due to an accumulation of fluid in the abdomen.

    ❑ True   ❑ False

12. It is recommended that children spend 60 minutes a day engaged in physical activity.

    ❑ True   ❑ False

Fill in the Blank

1. In toddlerhood, the period of decreased appetite as a result of decreased caloric need is often referred to as a time of _____.

2. The three major psychosocial tasks of toddlerhood are _____, _____, and _____.

3. The expressed need of the toddler to maintain sameness, such as using the same dish and cup, is called _____.

4. _____ are outward explosive reactions to inward stressful or frustrating situations that are a normal part of toddler life.

5. The average toddler is ready to begin toilet training at approximately _____ months.

6. Toddlers most often play alongside, but not with, other children. This type of play is called _____.

7. Examples of foods to avoid in toddlerhood that may be a major choking hazard include _____, _____, and _____.

8. The only type of balloon recommended as safe for young children is _____.

9. _____ is defined as intense feelings of jealousy between siblings, often seen when an infant is born into a family with a toddler.

Matching

_____ 1. temper tantrum

_____ 2. ritualism

_____ 3. physiologic anorexia

a. period of decreased appetite as a result of decreased caloric need

b. outward explosive reaction to inward stressful situation

c. need to maintain sameness

Multiple Choice

1. Dawn asks the nurse at what age she should expect her daughter to show signs of readiness to start toilet training. The best response by the nurse is:

   a. 12 months
   b. 15 months
   c. 24 months
   d. 36 months

2. At what age are most toddlers able to name body parts, give their full name, use about 900 different words, and speak in three- to five-word sentences?

   a. 12–15 months
   b. 18 months
   c. 24 months
   d. 36 months

3. Which one of the following actions is an acceptable method of disciplining the toddler?

   a. Communicate limits to the child.
   b. Inform the child that he or she is bad when the child does not follow the rules.
   c. Do not allow the child to test the limits.
   d. Teach the child to suppress undesirable feelings.

4. David is the father of 28-month-old Veronica. She has been throwing temper tantrums for the past two weeks. David asks the nurse why his daughter acts this way and what he can do about the situation. The best response by the nurse is:

   a. You must stop Veronica from having temper tantrums. If you don't stop them, she will be a spoiled, uncontrollable child.

   b. If Veronica holds her breath during the tantrum, it is usually harmless.

   c. After the tantrum is over, be sure to discipline Veronica for this unacceptable behavior.

   d. You can expect the temper tantrums to disappear by 6 years of age.

5. Which of the following statements will the nurse include when providing a talk on toilet training?

   a. Bowel control is often more difficult to attain than bladder control.

   b. Consistent day and night dryness should be achieved by 4 years of age.

   c. Praise the child for each attempt whether successful or not.

   d. The average child is ready to begin toilet training at 16–18 months of age.

6. Which of the following statements made by a caregiver of a toddler regarding play in this age group indicates further teaching is necessary?

   a. Children in the age group often play alongside, but not with, other children.

   b. It is normal for toddlers to demonstrate little attention to the feelings of play partners, and they frequently grab desired toys or hit others to keep a favorite toy.

   c. When a new toy is introduced into the toddlers' world, teach them how to use the toy.

   d. Toddlers should not be allowed to engage in make-believe, pretend, or fantasy play, as this will distort their perception of reality.

7. Ming-Li asks the nurse, "Juyong is hardly eating anything. He used to eat really well, but now that he is 2, I just can't get him to eat a good meal." What information should the nurse provide Ming-Li?

   a. Do not allow Juyong to eat between meals. Snacking will limit the amount of food he eats at meals.

   b. A general rule of thumb is to offer a quarter of a cup of food for each year.

   c. Encourage Juyong to participate in meal preparation.

   d. Allow Juyong to watch TV while eating his meals.

8. Which one of the following statements should be included in the teaching plan regarding dental health of the toddler?

    a. Use at least one inch of fluoridated toothpaste on the brush.

    b. Select a toothbrush with hard, long bristles.

    c. After cleansing the teeth, flossing is recommended.

    d. Purchase flavored fluoridated toothpaste to encourage the child to swallow and thus increase fluoride consumption.

9. The nurse observes the interaction of a caregiver with a toddler. Which of the following requires intervention by the nurse? The caregiver:

    a. uses food as a reward when the toddler cooperates

    b. positions self at the child's eye-level before speaking

    c. remembers that the child's attention span is approximately one minute per year of age

    d. relates time and scheduled events to familiar occurrences such as "after lunch"

10. Rahisha, who is the mother of a 25-month-old girl, tells the nurse, "My baby Jaquina is such a picky eater. I can hardly get her to eat anything at all. What can I do about this?" The best response by the nurse would be:

    a. Set a time limit for Jaquina and tell her that she will need to eat her food in ten minutes or she will be punished.

    b. Do not allow Jaquina to have food jags in which she eats the same food for more than two days; if you do, her picky eating will only get worse.

    c. Do not allow Jaquina to participate in meal preparation as seeing the food most likely takes her appetite away.

    d. Provide healthy snacks every one to two hours and keep them in a place where Jaquina can independently reach them.

Multiple Response

1. Maura tells the nurse, "My daughter Stephanie is 23 months old and so negative. Whenever I talk to her and ask her to do something, she always says no. What can I do about this? I don't want her to be so negative at such a young age." Which of the following responses by the nurse are appropriate? Select all that apply.

    a. Reduce the opportunity to say no by not giving Stephanie the option of saying no when you want her to do something.

    b. When Stephanie is tired or hungry, give her some quiet time and feed her rather than taking her out shopping or to visit with others.

    c. If Stephanie says no and acts up in public, wait until you are home with her and alone to discuss her behavior.

    d. When you want Stephanie to do something, tell her what the disciplinary guidelines are in brief and simple terms.

    e. Tell Stephanie she will not get a bike when she is 4.

    f. Develop a chart to show Stephanie which indicates when she has demonstrated unacceptable behavior.

2. Liandra tells the nurse, "My son Thomaso is 28 months old. He is so stubborn. Thomaso has to have the same breakfast, the same way, the same time every day. If he is this controlling now, what will he be like when he gets older? I don't know how to handle this." How should the nurse reply? Select all that apply.

    a. You must let Thomaso know who is in control early on or you can expect to have much difficulty with him as a teenager.

    b. You need to incorporate Thomaso's rituals into both of your lifestyles because rituals provide repetition through which he will gain comfort and security.

    c. Routines will allow Thomaso to master new skills while providing a sense of control over the environment.

    d. Thomaso is not stubborn; at this age rituals are his way to ask for his needs to be met.

    e. You and your son need professional help.

    f. The relationship you have with Thomaso in relation to power is determined now.

3. Tyler, age 26 months, has been admitted to the hospital for dehydration. When disciplining Tyler, the nurse should do which of the following? Select all that apply.

   a. Discuss with the caregivers how to support their method of discipline when Tyler is hospitalized.

   b. Explain to the caregivers that hospitalized children frequently display regressive behaviors and that everyone involved in his care should carefully think before implementing any disciplinary measures related to regressive behavior.

   c. Use the same method of physical punishment the caregivers use in the home.

   d. Follow discipline with love and positive encouragement.

   e. Do not allow Tyler to see his family if he misbehaves.

   f. Develop a new set of disciplinary actions to follow for the duration of his hospitalization.

4. Shaniqua is the mother of 2-year-old Do'nelle and 2-week-old DeWayne. Shaniqua tells the nurse, "Do'nelle is so jealous of the baby. She really doesn't like her brother and wants all of my attention. I need time to spend with DeWayne. What can I do?" What information should the nurse include when teaching Shaniqua about sibling rivalry? Select all that apply.

   a. Start to toilet train Do'nelle.

   b. Make Do'nelle give DeWayne one of her favorite toys.

   c. Establish a time frame when attention is focused exclusively on Do'nelle.

   d. Tell Do'nelle that DeWayne is her new playmate and encourage them to spend more time together.

   e. Encourage Do'nelle to participate in the care of DeWayne and praise positive interactions.

   f. Maintain Do'nelle's rituals as long as needed.

Critical Thinking/Case Study

A group of nursing students is on rotation at the neighborhood nursing center. Their clinical instructor has assigned them a project related to injury prevention in toddlers. The group has decided to make posters that will be displayed at the center. Help the group design the posters by answering the following questions.

1. What developmental characteristics of toddlers should the students consider?

    _____

    _____

    _____

2. What information should be included on the poster related to preventing injuries from motor vehicle accidents?

    _____

    _____

    _____

3. Preventing fall-related injuries?

    _____

    _____

    _____

4. Preventing aspiration?

    _____

    _____

    _____

5. Preventing suffocation?

    _____

    _____

    _____

6. Preventing burns?

_____

_____

_____

7. Preventing ingestion/poisoning?

_____

_____

_____

8. Promoting gun safety?

_____

_____

_____

9. Preventing drowning?

_____

_____

_____

10. Miscellaneous areas to promote safety?

_____

_____

_____

CHAPTER 10

Growth and Development of the Preschooler

True or False

1. During the preschool years, the rate of physical growth increases as compared to the rate experienced during the infant and toddler years.

   ❏ True   ❏ False

2. The preschool period is a time of refinement of eye-hand coordination and muscle coordination.

   ❏ True   ❏ False

3. The preschool years are characterized as a time when the child experiences intense attraction and love for the parent of the opposite sex.

   ❏ True   ❏ False

4. The chief psychosocial task of preschoolers described by Erikson is the development of a sense of initiative versus guilt.

   ❏ True   ❏ False

5. Sleep disturbances associated with the preschool years diminish as the child matures.

   ❏ True   ❏ False

6. Preschoolers cannot differentiate between reality and fantasy.

   ❏ True   ❏ False

Fill in the Blank

1. _____ is the capacity to understand and use phenomena in the world around us.

2. According to Piaget, the stage when the child develops the ability to perform mental operations governed by personal perceptions and linkage to events previously experienced is referred to as the _____ stage.

3. During the preschool years, the child is curious about his or her body and learns about the physical differences between boys and girls. Freud described this period of time as the _____ or _____ stage of psychosexual development.

4. Sentences that are three to four words in length are referred to as _____ speech. It is commonly found in _____-year-olds.

5. The child's conscience is also known as the _____.

6. According to Kohlberg, children of preschool age are in the _____ or _____ stage of moral development.

7. The American Academy of Pediatrics recommends a preschooler watch no more than _____ to _____ hours of television per day.

Matching

_____ 1. lordosis

_____ 2. animism

_____ 3. Oedipal complex

_____ 4. cognitive ability

_____ 5. Electra complex

a. a preschool boy's love for his mother

b. capacity to understand and use phenomena in the world

c. concave lumbar spine

d. belief that objects have human characteristics

e. a preschool girl's love for her father

Multiple Choice

1. Latoya asks the nurse what she can do about her preschool-age son not wanting to sleep as much as he has in the past. Latoya tells the nurse, "My son used to sleep so much until he turned 3 years old. I can hardly get anything done and he doesn't want to go to bed at night. What should I do?" Which of the following is the appropriate response for the nurse to make?

   a. Generally preschoolers sleep a total of 16 hours every day.
   b. There must be something wrong with your son. Maybe he has hyperactivity disorder.
   c. It is very important for you to establish a bedtime routine for your child.
   d. It would be best for you to let your son sleep and stay awake upon his individual demands.

2. When working with preschool children, the nurse identifies which age group as enjoying pretend play and "dress-up?"

   a. 2-year-olds

   b. 3-year-olds

   c. 4-year-olds

   d. 5-year-olds

3. A nurse performs a physical examination on a 4-year-old. Which of the following findings should the nurse report to the primary care provider?

   a. heart rate 108

   b. respiratory rate 12

   c. weight 37 pounds (16.7 kg)

   d. lordosis of the spine

4. A 4-year-old is admitted to the emergency department for evaluation after he fell off of his bike while riding down a hill. The child states, "The bike threw me off of it!" This is an example of:

   a. egocentrism

   b. transductive reasoning

   c. animism

   d. idiosyncratic reasoning

Multiple Response

1. Savannah asks the nurse what she should feed her preschool-age daughter to ensure proper nutrition. Which of the following should the nurse include in teaching? Select all that apply.

   a. Your daughter should start to eat table food by 4 years of age.

   b. The diet of a preschool child should revolve around the principles of the USDA's MyPyramid.

   c. The preschool child should be switched from drinking whole milk to low-fat or skim milk.

   d. A preschool child should be served one tablespoon of food per every year of age.

   e. Preschoolers need iron supplements with every meal.

   f. Include foods that are high in salt because 4-year-olds perspire a lot and you do not want their sodium levels to fall.

2. Keisha is a 4-year-old girl who weighs 80 pounds. Her mother tells the nurse she is proud of the fact that Keisha is a good eater and that at age 4, all of the baby fat Keisha has will go away with time. The nurse informs Keisha's mother that which of the following are complications of childhood obesity? Select all that apply.

   a. hyperlipidemia
   b. cerebral palsy
   c. obstructive apnea
   d. pancreatitis
   e. hypertension
   f. autism

3. Which of the following statements about the dental hygiene needs of preschool children will the nurse include in family education? Select all that apply.

   a. Tell the child he or she will experience no pain when visiting the dentist.
   b. If toothpaste contains fluoride, use a pea-sized amount.
   c. The child should visit the dentist at least every six months.
   d. Preschoolers should floss.
   e. Preschoolers should brush their teeth once a day.
   f. Preschoolers should use their index finger to brush their teeth.

4. Chronic low-level lead exposure in children causes which of the following? Select all that apply.

   a. impaired growth
   b. pica
   c. anemia
   d. hearing loss
   e. asthma
   f. attention-deficit disorder

Critical Thinking/Case Study

Towanda is a nurse working in a neighborhood wellness center. She would like to evaluate preschool children who visit the center and assess their physiologic development.

1. What standardized assessment tool can she use to accomplish this goal?

   _____

   _____

   _____

2. What can Towanda expect to find as "normal" height and weight increases between children ages 3, 4, and 5?

   _____

   _____

   _____

3. How does visual acuity change among these age groups?

   _____

   _____

   _____

4. What would be the best way for Towanda to assess gross motor development of these children?

   _____

   _____

   _____

5. How does gross motor development differ in the 3-, 4-, and 5-year-old?

   _____

   _____

   _____

6. What would be the best way for Towanda to assess fine motor development of these children?

_____

_____

_____

7. How does fine motor development differ between 3-, 4-, and 5-year-olds?

_____

_____

_____

8. When working with these children, how does the cognitive development differ between 3-, 4-, and 5-year-olds?

_____

_____

_____

9. What impact if any does this have on Towanda's interaction with these children?

_____

_____

_____

CHAPTER 11

Growth and Development of the School-Age Child

True or False

1. Growing pains are common in the school-age child because the long bones grow faster than the attached muscles.

   ❑ True   ❑ False

2. The peak incidence of growing pain is between the ages of 8 to 12 years.

   ❑ True   ❑ False

3. Although obesity occurs in all populations, its prevalence is pronounced among minority children.

   ❑ True   ❑ False

4. School-age boys and girls have the same number of muscle cells.

   ❑ True   ❑ False

5. As many as 50 percent of all school-age children between 6 and 10 years of age have an "innocent" heart murmur.

   ❑ True   ❑ False

6. The school-age years are often considered one of the healthiest phases of life.

   ❑ True   ❑ False

7. Piaget suggested that at around 6 years of age, children start to move from the flexible thought of the preschool age to the more egocentric view of the school-age child.

   ❑ True   ❑ False

8. According to Kohlberg, the school-age child is at the conventional level of moral development when the conscience develops an internal set of rules that must be followed in order to "be good."

   ❑ True   ❑ False

9. Athletic activities for the school-age child must be carefully selected because the child at this age has muscles and bones that are easily injured due to immaturity.

   ❑ True   ❑ False

10. The leading cause of death in the school-age child is accidents.

   ❑ True   ❑ False

Fill in the Blank

1. The six basic gross motor skills that continue to be refined in the school-age child are _____, _____, _____, _____, _____, and _____.

2. The average apical pulse rate for the school-age child is _____ beats per minute while at rest, and the average respiratory rate for the school-age child is _____ breaths per minute while at rest.

3. The average age for puberty in the United States is _____ years of age for females and _____ years of age for males.

4. According to Freud, starting at age 6 years and throughout school-age, the child enters a calm period in the development of sexuality called _____.

5. Erik Erikson identified the major task of the school-age period as _____ versus _____.

6. Sleep walking, otherwise known as _____, occurs in 15 percent of all school-age children and is not uncommon between 4 and 8 years of age.

7. Sleep talking, or _____, can occur at any age across the life span and does not indicate a health concern or need for intervention.

8. Inflicting verbal or physical harm on another is known as _____.

Matching

____ 1. conservation

____ 2. menarche

____ 3. malocclusion

____ 4. puberty

a. abnormality of the coming together of the teeth

b. appearance of secondary sex characteristics and the ability to reproduce

c. change in shape not change of amount

d. female's first period

Multiple Choice

1. Which one of the following is a school-age milestone of social development expected in the 6- to 7-year-old child?

    a. desires more independence
    b. develops interest in the opposite sex
    c. able to bathe and dress self
    d. increased interest in family

2. Which of the following is an accurate statement regarding sleep and rest in the school-age child?

    a. Most children at 6 years of age require eight to nine hours of sleep.
    b. Most children at 12 years of age require at least 10 hours of sleep.
    c. Most school-age children need to nap.
    d. Sleep is essential during the school-age years to foster physical growth and academic performance.

3. Tamara, age 9, is scheduled to have her tonsils removed. The best time for the nurse to provide preoperative education for her is:

    a. the morning of the surgery
    b. the afternoon before the surgery
    c. two days before the surgery
    d. one week before the surgery

4. Which statement by the caregiver of a school-age child indicates that more education on seat belt safety is indicated?

    a. Children age 6 years and older should sit in the front seat of the vehicle.
    b. Do not allow children to sit in the cargo area of pickup trucks.
    c. Correct seat belt fit is usually not achieved until the child is 9 years old.
    d. Seat belts fit correctly when the lap portion of the belt rides low over the hips.

Multiple Response

1. Rudy is a 9-year-old boy. His mother asks the nurse why he wakes up at night with cramps in his legs and what can be done to help him. Which of the following will the nurse include in the response? Select all that apply.

   a. Having Rudy wear shoes that are sturdy and supportive can be helpful.
   b. The discomfort is usually located in the knees, calves, and thighs.
   c. A warm bath can be used as a comfort measure.
   d. Growing pains are temporary and caused by muscles growing faster than bones.
   e. Mild analgesics have been found to be effective.
   f. Gentle massage to the legs has been found to be effective.

2. Santo, age 8, has been diagnosed with an innocent heart murmur. His father asks the nurse what this means and what can be done to help Santo. The nurse will share which information with the father? Select all that apply.

   a. Only about 10 percent of all school-age children have an innocent heart murmur.
   b. Murmurs are usually found between 6 and 10 years of age.
   c. The murmur will no longer be heard when the child reaches adolescence.
   d. The sound of the murmur is created from the blood flowing through the heart and can be heard because of the child's thin chest wall.
   e. The murmur is associated with the development of heart disease as an adult.
   f. If the murmur is present when Santo returns for a follow-up visit in 3 months, surgery will be scheduled.

3. According to Piaget, the expanded cognitive abilities of the school-age child include which of the following? Select all that apply.

   a. industry
   b. abstractism
   c. reversibility
   d. substitution
   e. classification
   f. conservation

4. Shaquille is a 10-year-old boy who has seen the school nurse multiple times for vague complaints. He tells the nurse he is being bullied by some of the older boys in the school. Which of the following signs or symptoms have been reported by children in response to bullying? Select all that apply.

   a. sleep disturbance
   b. fever
   c. headache
   d. stomachache
   e. sweating palms
   f. dizziness

Critical Thinking/Case Study

A large group of immigrants has become part of the community where a school nurse is practicing at the elementary level. A language barrier exists with these individuals. Most of the families are on public assistance until they are able to settle into their new environment. The nurse has been asked by the local health department to provide health education to the caregivers of the school-age children. Because accidents are the leading cause of death in this age group, the nurse decides to focus the first component of the series of talks on safety issues.

1. Where should the classes take place?

   _____

   _____

   _____

2. What time should the nurse hold the classes?

   _____

   _____

   _____

3. How can the nurse deal with the language barrier that exists?

   _____

   _____

   _____

4. Prioritize the safety issues the nurse should discuss with this group.

   _____

   _____

   _____

5. What teaching methods should be utilized? Handouts? Posters?

   _____

   _____

   _____

6. Summarize components of safety teaching the nurse will include for: motor vehicles, bikes, skateboards, roller blades, trampolines, pedestrians, swimming, firearms, strangers, drug use, smoking, and medicines.

   _____

   _____

   _____

7. What would be the best method to use in assessing the cultural similarities and differences between the nurse and the participants?

   _____

   _____

   _____

CHAPTER 12

Growth and Development of the Adolescent

True or False

1. Adolescence is second only to infancy in relation to the amount of change individuals encounter physiologically and psychosocially.

   ❑ True   ❑ False

2. The concept of an adolescent stage of development is a relatively recent phenomenon, having been recognized in the beginning of the 20th century.

   ❑ True   ❑ False

3. Gender differences in skeletal growth patterns of adolescents include females having greater arm and leg length relative to trunk size, and delayed skeletal ossification when compared with males.

   ❑ True   ❑ False

4. The heart almost doubles in weight and increases in size by about one half during adolescence.

   ❑ True   ❑ False

5. According to Selman, the cognitive reasoning of the adolescent focuses on the importance of the self in social interactionalism.

   ❑ True   ❑ False

6. According to Erikson, the major crisis of adolescence is establishing relationships.

   ❑ True   ❑ False

7. Because of the psychosocial development of adolescents, the concern for moral values and standards is likely to never be more relevant than during adolescence.

   ❑ True   ❑ False

8. Adolescents' attachment to caregivers is important and has been linked to such characteristics as self-esteem and emotional adjustment.

   ❑ True   ❑ False

9. Conflict between caregivers and adolescents most often centers around "hot" issues such as sex, drugs, religion, or politics.

   ❑ True   ❑ False

10. Adolescents experiencing divorce exhibit slightly lower levels of well-being than adolescents from continuously intact families.

    ❑ True   ❑ False

11. For most adolescents, ethnicity or culture appears to be very important in determining whom they select as friends.

    ❑ True   ❑ False

12. Adolescents who exist at the periphery of their peer group would be most vulnerable to peer influence as a result of their insecure position in the group.

    ❑ True   ❑ False

13. Although fully developed in size, the brain actually continues to change in numerous ways during adolescence.

    ❑ True   ❑ False

14. From a psychoanalytical perspective, moral development of adolescents arises out of the individual's fear of rejection as a result of his or her inability to control unconscious impulses.

    ❑ True   ❑ False

Fill in the Blank

1. Adolescence consists of three relatively distinct periods: _____ or _____, _____ or _____, and _____ or _____.

2. _____ is the state of physical development when secondary sex characteristics begin to appear, sexual organs mature, reproduction first becomes possible, and the adolescent growth spurt starts. _____, on the other hand, is that time of life that begins with puberty and ends when the individual is physically and psychologically mature and able to assume adult responsibilities.

3. Before puberty, the primary hormone regulating growth is _____.

4. During the adolescent growth spurt, the male typically gains _____ pounds and grows _____ inches. Females typically gain _____ pounds and grow _____ inches.

5. In the adolescent female, estrogen causes breast changes including _____, _____ of the reproductive organs, and growth/darkening of the _____ and _____ hair.

6. In adolescent males, follicle-stimulating hormone is responsible for _____ and _____. Luteinizing hormone promotes _____ and _____ production.

7. In females, the first menstrual period is known as _____.

8. The transient breast enlargement experienced by some adolescent males is called _____.

9. According to Elkind, _____ is when one is unable to appropriately differentiate between oneself and one's objects of attention.

10. A major task for adolescents is answering the questions, _____, and _____.

11. Peer relationships of adolescents generally exist at one of three levels: _____, or coming together of two friends; _____, a group of three to nine "buddies" who exhibit a strong sense of cohesion; and _____, an association of two to four cliques in which relations are less intimate than in the smaller groups.

12. Common issues related to nutrition that surface during the nutritional assessment of the adolescent include _____, _____, and_____.

13. Three major environmental factors that are thought to be related to genetics and contribute to rising obesity rates of adolescents include _____, _____, and _____.

14. Numerous hazards of alcohol ingestion in the adolescent include: _____, _____, _____, _____, _____, _____, _____, _____, _____, _____, _____, and _____.

Matching

_____ 1. Vygotsky

_____ 2. clique

_____ 3. moratorium

_____ 4. egocentrism

_____ 5. pubertal

_____ 6. Kohlberg

_____ 7. Elkind

_____ 8. Tanner stages

_____ 9. gynecomastia

a. small group of peers who regularly interact with one another

b. inability to appreciate the differences in oneself and the objects of one's attention

c. middle adolescence

d. zone of proximal development

e. imaginary audience and personal fable

f. exploration of questions, occupations, or ideologic choices with no firm set of commitments

g. transient breast enlargement

h. sequence of secondary sexual characteristics

i. Moral theory

Multiple Choice

1. When performing a physical assessment on a preadolescent female, the nurse identifies which of the following as the first visible sign of female sexual maturation?

   a. menstruation
   b. growth of pubic hair
   c. breast development
   d. enlargement of the labia

2. The average age of menarche is:

   a. 8 years of age
   b. 10 years of age
   c. 12 years of age
   d. 14 years of age

3. Which of the developmental theorists viewed adolescence and physical changes of puberty as reawakening the sexual and aggressive energies felt toward parents during early childhood, resulting in detachment from parents?

   a. Erikson
   b. Piaget
   c. Brenner
   d. Freud

4. According to Piaget's stage of formal operations, the most distinct feature of adolescents' thinking is that they:

   a. can consider what is possible, rather than what is real
   b. focus on the physical world of their existence
   c. base potential solutions on previous experiences
   d. are not able to consider their own thoughts as real objects

5. According to Marcia, adolescents who demonstrate a strong sense of commitment but have not experienced a crisis or exploratory period necessary for arriving at their sense of commitment are taking the following path to identity status:

   a. identity achievement
   b. foreclosure
   c. identity diffusion
   d. moratorium

6. A nurse working with an adolescent reared in an authoritarian home would expect the adolescent to most likely:

   a. be more dependent and passive
   b. act more irresponsibly and be less able to assume leadership positions
   c. be more impulsive and more likely to be involved in delinquent behavior
   d. act more responsibly and be self-assured and creative

7. A nurse is asked by a group of parents of adolescents to provide a talk on peer relationships of adolescents. The nurse will include which one of the following statements in her talk?

   a. There is usually considerable overlap between parental and peer values because of common backgrounds; many adolescents select friends whose values are congruent with those of their parents.

   b. Peers are more likely than parents to be influential in matters of great and long-term permanence such as moral and social values, educational aspirations, and occupational choice.

   c. Adolescents turn to peers for support because of displacement of parental influence.

   d. As parents you are advised to control your child's peer relations to ensure the proper influence for your child.

8. When working with adolescents, which of the following statements would be suggested by the nurse to ease the transition for students going from elementary to middle school or high school?

   a. You can expect the class to be about the same. A homeroom teacher will teach all of the subjects. Don't worry, you're going to a different building; not much else will change.

   b. You can expect to work in groups most of the time with your teachers providing opportunities for you to learn for the sake of learning in a very relaxed atmosphere.

   c. Be prepared for a complex classroom organization with a faster-paced curriculum. You can expect the teachers to focus on discipline as an important component of the educational experience.

   d. You can expect to be in an environment that fosters your autonomy.

9. Fredrick is a 17-year-old who has had a drastic change in his attitude, appearance, and school performance. Fredrick exhibits irrational behavior; preoccupation with the occult; decreased quality of schoolwork; irresponsibility; changes in personality, friends, activities, and appearance; difficulty communicating; rebelliousness; mental and physiologic deterioration; and unexplainable loss of money. The nurse suspects that Fredrick is most likely experiencing:

   a. depression caused by fear of adult commitments

   b. drug abuse of some form

   c. anorexia nervosa

   d. a dramatic effort to rebel against adult conformity

Multiple Response

1. When working with adolescents, the nurse needs to be aware that sense of identity for the adolescent is based on primary factors in his or her life, including which of the following? Select all that apply.

   a. individual identification established during childhood
   b. how well he or she is doing in school at the present time
   c. the adolescent's ability to master each developmental task
   d. establishing his or her own ideology based on social attitudes adopted
   e. establishing his or her own ideology based on political attitudes adopted
   f. establishing his or her own ideology based on religious attitudes adopted

2. General nursing interactions that should be used to foster health promotion in the adolescent include which of the following? Select all that apply.

   a. Provide an environment that is caring.
   b. Treat adolescents with dignity.
   c. Perform assessments that focus on improving health, and describe health-promoting behaviors.
   d. Maintain a trusting relationship with adolescents.
   e. Get to know the adolescent as an individual.
   f. Do not inform family of any interactions with adolescents.

3. A mother of a 13-year-old boy asks the nurse what she should provide as food sources for her son: "I can't believe how much Andrew's appetite has increased over the past few weeks. He is eating all of the time. What can you tell me about the dietary needs of an adolescent?" What information should the nurse share? Select all that apply.

   a. Calcium is needed to meet skeletal growth requirements and to prevent fractures.
   b. Zinc is necessary for final body growth and sexual maturation.
   c. You do not need to worry about increasing iron sources because Andrew will not menstruate.
   d. Andrew needs caloric content of about 2,500 to 3,000 calories per day.
   e. Protein intake should be increased.
   f. It is normal for an adolescent to always seem hungry.

Critical Thinking/Case Study

The nurse enters a room of a health center to find an elderly woman with her granddaughter. The grandmother says, "I need you to help my granddaughter. Look how fat she is. I have tried everything, but all she does is eat. I don't want to be mean, but she has to do something and we need your help." The nurse continues the conversation and performs an assessment with the following data obtained.

The girl's name is Selma. She is 14 years old. Selma is 5 feet 2 inches tall and weighs 218 pounds. Selma has had her menstrual period on an irregular basis for the past two years. She frequently has very heavy days followed by periods of light flow days. Her blood pressure is up at 182/96. Selma states that she does not go out with her friends much because she basically does not have many friends. "Everyone makes fun of me; they call me fat girl." When asked about activity, Selma states that she hates gym class because she is always out of breath and sweating. "I don't play any sports; I stink at everything I try to do." Selma tells the nurse, "I want to be normal. I can't even buy clothes in stores for kids my age. I have to go to the fat lady stores, and everyone makes fun of how I look. Please help me."

1. Is Selma ready to be taught about health promotion behaviors?

   _____

   _____

   _____

2. What are some of the nursing diagnoses according to North American Nursing Diagnosis Association (NANDA) that the nurse can identify based on the assessment?

   _____

   _____

   _____

3. What would be the best way to obtain a diet history on Selma?

   _____

   _____

   _____

4. What would the nurse assess Selma's body image to be?

_____

_____

_____

5. Why is body image such an important component to the well-being of the adolescent?

_____

_____

_____

CHAPTER 13

Child and Family Communication

True or False

1. Communication is defined as the exchange of meanings between and among individuals through a shared system of symbols.

   ❑ True   ❑ False

2. Communication consists of talking and listening.

   ❑ True   ❑ False

3. To establish rapport, the nurse should address the family members of the child by their first names to convey a sense of trust.

   ❑ True   ❑ False

4. Therapeutic relationships should be caring and empathetic, but should avoid emotional involvement and overprotectiveness.

   ❑ True   ❑ False

5. When engaged in conversation with a child or his or her family, it is imperative that the nurse maintain eye contact and expect to receive eye contact from the child and family at all times.

   ❑ True   ❑ False

6. Humor is healing and can bridge communicative gaps even when the direct communication is feared or offensive; it is recognized as an effective method of assisting children and adolescents to cope with illness, pain, and hospitalization.

   ❑ True   ❑ False

7. Writing is an especially effective method of communicating with older school-age children and adolescents.

   ❑ True   ❑ False

8. Cultural background can play a role in determining an individual's communication pattern.

   ❏ True   ❏ False

9. Infancy is a time when communication is achieved through nonverbal means.

   ❏ True   ❏ False

10. The communication pattern of the Japanese culture consists of much touching and embracing to communicate feelings.

    ❏ True   ❏ False

Fill in the Blank

1. The major components of the communication process are the _____, _____, _____, _____, and _____.

2. Some physical or environmental barriers to communication include: _____, _____, _____, _____, _____, and _____.

3. Psychosocial barriers to communication include: _____, _____, _____, _____, _____, and _____.

4. _____ refers to communication that occurs in an organized way, with a particular agenda, as when teaching a child's care to the caregiver upon discharge. _____ occurs when individuals talk using no particular agenda or protocol.

5. Paraverbal cues, also part of verbal communication, include _____, _____, _____, _____, and _____.

6. Before communication can be effective, several key elements must be addressed, including _____, _____, _____, _____, _____, _____, _____, and _____.

7. _____ refers to the ability to put oneself in the other person's shoes—to feel as well as to intellectually know what the other person is experiencing.

8. The four Bs of effective listening are _____, _____, _____, and _____.

Matching

_____ 1. touch

_____ 2. channel

_____ 3. empathy

a. ability to put one's self in the other person's shoes

b. medium through which a message is transmitted

c. kinesthetic channel

Multiple Choice

1. In which one of the following situations is the nurse interacting with the child and family in an empathetic manner?

   a. The nurse feels sorry for the child and family.

   b. The nurse offers condolence and pity to the child and family.

   c. The nurse assumes all of the child's care.

   d. The nurse maintains a sense of objectivity and gives examples of facilitating the child's and parent's ability to function in difficult and sad situations.

2. The nurse who practices within professional boundaries established in relationships with the child and family will:

   a. socialize with the child and family

   b. assist the parents in caring for and nurturing their child

   c. accept gifts offered by the caregiver and child

   d. share personal information such as a home telephone number

3. When providing care to a 4-month-old infant, the nurse uses effective communication with the baby by:

   a. removing the caregivers from the environment when interacting with the child to avoid distraction

   b. completing all tasks quickly to avoid overstimulation of the baby

   c. gently rubbing or patting the infant while securely holding him or her

   d. using verbal communication methods at all times, as this is the most effective method of communication with infants

4. Which one of the following statements is true regarding communication with toddlers?

   a. Wordy explanations of procedures should be given to the toddler.

   b. Explain procedures to the toddler well in advance.

   c. Use play or books to demonstrate or describe activities or procedures.

   d. Most communication with the child should be nonverbal.

5. Communication with preschoolers can be enhanced by the nurse when which one of the following is done?

   a. allowing the child to make choices when possible

   b. telling the child that a painful procedure will not hurt so the child will cooperate

   c. removing equipment from the environment before the procedure so the child will not be afraid of what is to occur

   d. explaining to the child how a "good boy" or "good girl" should act

6. A nurse is presenting a talk on conflict resolution to a group of parents. The nurse should stress that which of the following is the most important first step to take to achieve resolution through communication?

   a. generate alternative solutions together

   b. negotiate the solution

   c. actively listen to the child

   d. tell the child what to do

7. Sequoia, age 4 years, is scheduled to have tubes placed in her ears because of frequent ear infections. When would be the best time for the nurse to teach Sequoia about the procedure?

   a. right before the procedure is to be carried out

   b. 1–3 hours before the procedure

   c. several days in advance of the procedure

   d. up to one week prior to the experience

8. Communication with adolescents can be enhanced by the nurse via:

   a. realization that adolescents are not able to comprehend most adult concepts

   b. use of concrete examples, as adolescents are not able to understand hypothetical situations

   c. discouragement of conversations concerning trivial matters

   d. active listening without demonstration of surprise, disapproval, or trivialization of matters discussed by the adolescent

Multiple Response

1. When taking part in communication, the nurse is aware of the fact that verbal communication can be more effective if it is which of the following? Select all that apply.

   a. lengthy
   b. clear
   c. well timed
   d. paced
   e. respectful of silent periods
   f. takes into account nonverbal cues

2. The nurse is caring for a 4-year-old child who is in need of intravenous fluid to correct a problem of dehydration. To prepare the child for this procedure the nurse will do which of the following? Select all that apply.

   a. Offer choices only if they exist.
   b. Talk to the caregivers and have them relay information to the child.
   c. Provide honest answers.
   d. Position self so communication with the child is at eye level.
   e. Use story telling as a possible technique to relay information.
   f. Teach the child about the procedure the day before.

3. Which of the following are effective methods of communicating with school-age children? Select all that apply.

   a. explaining treatments immediately before they occur
   b. using videos to explain procedures
   c. promoting conversations that encourage critical thinking
   d. providing enhanced details of the procedure if requested by the child
   e. allowing the expression of fear
   f. providing adequate time to answer questions

4. Communication patterns of the Vietnamese culture include which of the following? Select all that apply.

   a. avoidance of direct eye contact
   b. rigid concept of time
   c. modesty of speech
   d. disrespectful to question authority figures
   e. valuing harmony
   f. respect for generational relationships

Critical Thinking/Case Study

The nurse is practicing in a community-based wellness center. Most of the clients who visit the center are Hispanic Americans (Mexican). The age range of clients varies from infancy to late adulthood. Some of the clients have been born and raised in the United States, while others have recently moved to the United States from Mexico and have not experienced an "American" culture.

1. When interacting with clients of this Hispanic American culture, which type of eye contact should be used by the nurse for the most effective method of communication?

   _____

   _____

   _____

2. Should touch be routinely used in communication efforts?

   _____

   _____

   _____

3. Which parent, if any, should be present when speaking with a male child?

   _____

   _____

   _____

4. If personal topics are discussed, does the gender of the nurse have any impact?

   _____

   _____

   _____

5. What is the most effective method to assess whether the individuals understand what has been discussed with them?

   _____

   _____

   _____

6. What is the most effective way to approach discussion of a serious topic? What types of questions should be asked?

   _____

   _____

   _____

7. What would be the most effective method of communicating with an infant of this culture?

   _____

   _____

   _____

8. How would the nurse communicate with a Hispanic-American toddler who is in need of a series of immunization injections?

   _____

   _____

   _____

9. A school-age Hispanic-American child visits the wellness center to learn about summer safety issues. How would the nurse best communicate with this child?

   _____

   _____

   _____

10. An adolescent female Hispanic-American client visits the wellness center with questions concerning methods of birth control. What would be the most effective way for the nurse to communicate with this young woman?

    _____

    _____

    _____

CHAPTER 14

Pediatric Assessment

True or False

1. Head circumference should be measured in all children under 2 years of age during the physical assessment.

   ❏ True   ❏ False

2. Honey should not be given to children less than 1 year of age secondary to the risk of botulism.

   ❏ True   ❏ False

3. The caregiver is encouraged to switch the child from whole to 2% milk at 1 year of age.

   ❏ True   ❏ False

4. Blood pressure and rectal temperature measurements should be performed toward the beginning of the assessment.

   ❏ True   ❏ False

5. It is best to observe expansion of the abdomen in infants and toddlers during the respiratory assessment.

   ❏ True   ❏ False

6. A radial pulse can be obtained in children at 1 year of age.

   ❏ True   ❏ False

7. The most important aspect of obtaining a blood pressure for a child is choosing the correct cuff size.

   ❏ True   ❏ False

8. Blood pressures can be palpated for the infant and toddler.

   ❏ True   ❏ False

9. A dark black tuft of hair or a dimple over the lumbosacral area is normal in the Asian population.

   ❏ True   ❏ False

10. By 2 months of age, the head of the infant should stay in line with the body when being pulled forward.

    ❏ True   ❏ False

11. Absence of deciduous teeth beyond 16 months of age signifies an abnormality most commonly related to genetic causes.

    ❏ True   ❏ False

12. By age 4, the chest attains the adult configuration of lateral diameter greater than the anterior-posterior diameter.

    ❏ True   ❏ False

13. Stridor is indicative of upper airway obstruction, particularly edema in children.

    ❏ True   ❏ False

14. Lordosis is abnormal after 6 years of age.

    ❏ True   ❏ False

15. Tools to assess childhood obesity and those children at risk are now completed at each yearly visit to a child's primary health care provider.

    ❏ True   ❏ False

16. During examination of the middle ear of an Asian child, the examiner may note tiny white flecks within the canal. This is considered to be a normal finding representing dead skin cells.

    ❏ True   ❏ False

Fill in the Blank

1. For the infant born prematurely, the nurse needs to adjust the chronological age on the growth chart. For instance, the correct age for an 8-month-old infant who was born two months prematurely would be _____ months.

2. Two methods to determine dietary intake include _____ and _____.

3. Two commonly ordered laboratory tests during a nutritional assessment include _____ and _____.

4. The task of measuring the human body as height, weight, and size of component parts, including skin folds, is referred to as _____.

5. A newborn whose growth has been retarded in utero is referred to as _____. A newborn weight greater than the _____ gestational age percentile is abnormal.

6. When performing an assessment of the eyes, the nurse notes that the eyes are looking downward and the sclera is visible above the iris. The nurse correctly documents this finding as _____.

7. Prominent locations for detecting cyanosis or jaundice in the child include _____, _____, _____, _____, and _____.

8. A positive Ortolani's sign consists of the child exhibiting _____, _____, _____, and _____.

9. Failure of the testis to descend into the scrotal sac is called _____.

10. The order of abdominal assessment is _____, _____, and _____.

11. The most widely used development screening tool for assessing neuromuscular development of a child from birth through 6 years of age is the _____.

12. A common skin lesion found on newborns identified at the time of examination is _____, commonly known as a stork bite.

Matching

____ 1. milia

____ 2. acrocyanosis

____ 3. vernix caseosa

____ 4. hydrocephalus

____ 5. telangiectatic nevi

____ 6. craniosynostosis

____ 7. cyanosis

a. dusky blue color

b. pediculosis capitis

c. premature ossification of suture lines

d. deep-blue to black pigmentation over the lumbar and sacral areas of the spine, over the buttocks, and sometimes over the upper back and shoulders

e. clubfoot

f. cradle cap

g. moles

_____ 8. head lice

_____ 9. caput succedaneum

_____ 10. Mongolian spot

_____ 11. pectus carinatum

_____ 12. nevi

_____ 13. genu valgum

_____ 14. seborrheic dermatitis

_____ 15. metatarsus varus

_____ 16. microcephaly

h. small white papules on cheeks, forehead, nose, and chin of the newborn

i. imbalance of cerebrospinal fluid production and reabsorption

j. thick, cheesy, protective, integumentary deposit of the newborn

k. bluish-purple color of hands and feet while rest of the body remains pink

l. swelling over the occipitoparietal region of the skull

m. small brain, small head, and mental deficit

n. pigeon chest

o. stork bites

p. knock-knee

Multiple Choice

1. The nurse wants to assess how much fluid a 2-month-old infant is receiving on a daily basis. The best question the nurse can ask to elicit this information is:

    a. How much weight has your baby gained since birth?
    b. How often does your baby drink a day?
    c. How many stools a day does your baby have?
    d. How many wet diapers does your baby have in a 24-hour period?

2. When performing an assessment on a child, the supervising nurse needs to intervene if the new nurse:

    a. allows the child to express feelings
    b. explains that will be done prior to each portion of the assessment
    c. assures the child that all components of the exam will be comfortable
    d. establishes a trusting relationship with the child

3. When performing a temperature assessment on a child, the nurse should:

    a. be cautious in obtaining a rectal temperature in children less than 2 years of age due to risk of rectal perforation

    b. use the oral route of temperature assessment for a 3-year-old

    c. obtain a rectal exam for a child experiencing diarrhea to obtain the most accurate reading

    d. report a body temperature of 39.8° C (103.64° F) as afebrile for a 6-year-old child

4. Depka's baby Hasari is 5 days old. Hasari developed jaundice when he was 3 days old. Depka asks the nurse why her baby has yellow skin. The best response by the nurse is:

    a. Hasari's skin is yellow because his kidneys are immature.

    b. Hasari's liver is not mature enough yet to remove a substance called bilirubin from his system.

    c. Hasari's skin is yellow because you must have had an infection when you were pregnant.

    d. Your blood type and Hasari's are incompatible; the yellow color will go away soon.

5. Which of the following statements is true regarding assessment of the fontanels of a 2-month-old infant?

    a. Place the infant in the supine position to assess the fontanels.

    b. A sunken, depressed fontanel indicates the infant has mental retardation.

    c. A bulging, tense fontanel indicates increased intracranial pressure.

    d. The anterior fontanel should be closed by 2 months of age.

6. A nurse is asked to speak with a client who has just delivered a baby who was delivered with forceps. The mother asks the nurse, "What is wrong with my baby's head? Is he sick? Why is there a bump on his head?" The most appropriate response by the nurse is:

    a. I don't know. You should ask the doctor.

    b. Your baby's head is too big.

    c. All babies are born with some bumps.

    d. Often during a forceps delivery, due to pressure, there is some slight bleeding in the area of the skull that causes a bump. It should resolve within a couple of weeks.

7. The nurse is assessing the tympanic membrane of a 2-year-old child. Which of the following would be considered a normal finding?

    a. pearly gray color
    b. opaque membrane
    c. fluid level behind the membrane
    d. dull light reflex

8. The nurse uses which of the following to assess for coarctation of the aorta?

    a. Palpate the carotid pulses simultaneously to assess for deficit.
    b. Palpate the brachial and femoral pulses simultaneously and assess for presence of brachial-femoral lag.
    c. Obtain blood pressure reading in the upper right arm and upper left arm, and compare results.
    d. Compare quality of radial and dorsalis pedis pulse.

9. The most effective general approach for assessment of the musculoskeletal system in a child is:

    a. Ask the child to perform specific activities.
    b. Observe the musculoskeletal system in the ambulatory child as the child moves freely about and plays in the exam room while the health history is being taken.
    c. Move through the assessment quickly to avoid boredom in the child.
    d. Start the process asking about the presence of muscle aches, as they are indicative of pathology in the child.

10. The nurse identifies which of the following as the expected normal respiratory rate of a newborn?

    a. 30–50
    b. 20–40
    c. 20–30
    d. 16–20

Multiple Response

1. Which of the following statements about assessment of the cervical lymph nodes of the infant are true? Select all that apply.

   a. Move the chin of the infant downward with hand before proceeding with palpation.
   b. Small, movable, cool, nontender nodes are referred to as "shotty" nodes.
   c. Enlargement of occipital nodes can occur in tinea capitis.
   d. Lymph nodes are generally not palpable.
   e. Use the finger pads to palpate lymph nodes.
   f. Use a circular motion when palpating lymph nodes.

2. When performing an examination of the genitalia of a pediatric female client, the nurse should follow which of the following procedures? Select all that apply.

   a. Ask the caregiver of an infant or young school-age child to leave the room.
   b. Drape the older-than-preschool-age child.
   c. Reserve the lithotomy position with the feet in stirrups for the older adolescent.
   d. Place the child older than 4 years on the examination table in a semilithotomy position without the feet in stirrups.
   e. Teach the child that it is not appropriate for anyone else to touch them in this manner.
   f. Explain what will be done before completing the examination.

Critical Thinking/Case Study

This morning the nurse is to perform complete physical assessments on four children: Afrom, a 4-month-old infant; Tung, a 3-year-old; Arlene, who is 9; and Jan, who is 14. The following questions focus on examination of the eye.

1. What is the general approach to the physical examination the nurse will use for each of the four children based on their developmental level?

   _____

   _____

   _____

2. Which children can be tested using the Snellen chart? The Snellen E chart? The Allen test?

_____

_____

_____

3. How will the nurse perform each test?

_____

_____

_____

4. How will the process used for testing differ for the children?

_____

_____

_____

5. Based on age, what are the normal and abnormal results for each test?

_____

_____

_____

6. Summarize the procedure the nurse will use for each child in obtaining the red reflex, evaluating the retina, and observing the optic disc.

_____

_____

_____

CHAPTER 15

Infectious Diseases

True or False

1. Children experience higher incidences of infectious diseases than adults because of an immature immune system and developmental and biologic variances.

   ❑ True   ❑ False

2. Virulence is the degree or power of a microorganism to cause disease.

   ❑ True   ❑ False

3. A reservoir is a place where pathogens can survive without multiplication.

   ❑ True   ❑ False

4. A carrier is a person who can harbor and spread an organism to others without becoming ill.

   ❑ True   ❑ False

5. The process of transmitting a disease from one generation to another is known as horizontal transmission.

   ❑ True   ❑ False

6. The diagnosis of giardia is made by the identification of cysts in fecal samples or enzyme immunoassay to detect *G. lamblia* antigens.

   ❑ True   ❑ False

7. The average infant who is immunized by the age of 2 according to current national guidelines will receive approximately 22 injections if each vaccine is given separately.

   ❑ True   ❑ False

8. Precautions must be taken when administering live vaccines such as measles, mumps, and rubella as well as varicella to adolescent girls and women of childbearing age to make certain that they are not pregnant at the time of vaccination.

   ❑ True   ❑ False

9. Hepatitis A is a disease that must be reported to the Centers for Disease Control and Prevention (CDC).

    ❏ True   ❏ False

10. Treatment of ascariasis includes mebendazole (Vermox) or pyrantel pamoate (Antiminth).

    ❏ True   ❏ False

11. A common sequela of chickenpox is viral encephalitis.

    ❏ True   ❏ False

12. Clinical manifestations of tetanus include headache and restlessness, followed by spasms of mastication muscles, difficulty opening mouth, dysphagia, and eventually opisthotonos, neck pain with bending, seizures, dysuria and urinary retention, bowel incontinence, and fever.

    ❏ True   ❏ False

Fill in the Blank

1. The discovery of _____ and the development of _____ has decreased the morbidity and mortality rates associated with most communicable and infectious diseases, particularly in industrialized countries.

2. _____ is any disease caused by growth of pathogenic microorganisms in the body. These diseases may or may not be contagious from person to person. _____ is an infectious disease that exhibits the potential to spread from person to person.

3. The seriousness of an infectious disease is dependent upon several factors, including _____, _____, _____, and _____.

4. The transmission of disease is dependent upon six factors that are referred to as the chain of infection. They include: _____, _____, _____, _____, _____, and _____.

5. Pathogens can also be transmitted on objects, in contaminated water or food, or by _____ (animals or insects that carry the infectious organism from one host to another).

6. _____ is the most common cause of sepsis, sinusitis, pneumonia, otitis media, and meningitis in children under the age of 2.

7. Mycobacterium tuberculosis, which includes new drug-resistant strains, has made a comeback and is especially devastating to those infected with the _____ virus.

8. The two permanent contraindications to vaccination are _____ and _____.

9. The earliest phase or sign of a developing condition or disease is known as the _____.

10. The infectious period for chickenpox is _____ days before the eruption of the rash to _____ days after the onset of the lesions when crusts have formed.

Matching

_____ 1. human papilloma virus

_____ 2. erythema infectiosum

_____ 3. teratogen

_____ 4. pathogen

_____ 5. pertussis

_____ 6. carrier

_____ 7. vector

_____ 8. varicella

_____ 9. virulence

_____ 10. tinea corporis

_____ 11. Reye's syndrome

a. disease-producing organisms

b. genital warts

c. whooping cough

d. ringworm of the body

e. Fifth's disease

f. persons harboring and spreading organisms without being ill

g. substance or process that interferes with normal prenatal development

h. encephalopathy and fatty degeneration of the liver

i. power of the microorganism to cause disease

j. chicken pox

k. animals or insects that carry infective organisms from one host to another

Multiple Choice

1. When talking with the supervisor of a day care center about prevention of the spread of infection, the nurse will need to intervene if the supervisor:

   a. discusses the importance of keeping immunizations up to date

   b. instructs personnel to wipe surface areas used for diaper changing with a disinfectant three times a day

   c. mentions a policy which states that staff must avoid changing diapers on rugs, upholstered furniture, and bed coverings

   d. states that when changing diapers, the staff members must wear gloves

2. A nurse is caring for a 3-month-old infant with an infection. The nurse recognizes which one of the following as the most common problem encountered by infants due to infection?

   a. dehydration

   b. anaphylaxis

   c. diabetes mellitus

   d. hypertension

3. Rita is the school nurse at a local elementary school. Her office is filled with children who have been sent to see her by their teachers. Which one of the following children will most likely be permitted to stay in school?

   a. Jack, age 9, who has diarrhea

   b. Bobby, age 7, who has a sore throat and no fever

   c. Leah, age 10, who has nits from head lice

   d. Andrew, age 11, who has purulent conjunctivitis

4. When reviewing requirements for current immunization, the nurse tells an expectant mother that at birth it is recommended that her baby receive which one of the following immunizations?

   a. varicella (var)

   b. measles, mumps, rubella (MMR)

   c. inactivated polio vaccine (IPV)

   d. hepatitis B (hep B)

5. Danielle, age 5, is ready to enter kindergarten. The state Danielle lives in requires children to be up to date in all immunizations before entering school. Susan, the nurse responsible to register children for entry to school, notices that Danielle has received only one hepatitis B vaccine at 2 months of age. Danielle's mom asks Susan what should be done. The best response by Susan is:

   a. Since Danielle had the vaccine so long ago, it has lost any effect in her system and the series of injections will need to be restarted.

   b. The series of injections will not need to be restarted. Make an appointment with your primary health care provider to have the series completed.

   c. Because Danielle has no risk factors for hepatitis B, she is exempt from the need to receive the immunizations.

   d. The remaining three doses of hepatitis B vaccines can be given to Danielle at the next appointment you make with your primary health care provider.

6. A mother of a 2-month-old infant is seen in the health clinic for a routine exam and scheduled immunizations. The mom asks the nurse, "Why does my baby need so many shots? I read that the shots can be given together so the baby does not have to suffer through so many needle sticks. What do you know about this?" Which of the following would be the best response by the nurse?

   a. You are absolutely right. Combination vaccination is the best way to go. There are no problems associated with the process.

   b. Some of the difficulties encountered with combination vaccines include febrile seizures associated with MMR combined vaccination.

   c. Combination of vaccinations does not have to be approved by the Food and Drug Administration (FDA); it is up to the primary care provider to decide whether it will be used.

   d. Combination vaccination requires the same immunization schedule as standard immunizations, so problems are avoided.

7. The father of a newborn has read about immunizations required for all children. He asks the nurse, "Why does my son need to have all of these shots? When I was a kid, the polio immunization was given by a sugar cube; it was a treat, not painful. Why should my son have to suffer through a shot? Besides there is no more polio." The best response by the nurse is:

    a. You are right about polio; it is not found anywhere on the planet. It is common practice to continue to administer it, however.

    b. There are no complications associated with administration of the polio vaccination, so don't worry about it.

    c. The oral preparation of polio vaccine (OPV) that you received as a child is capable of producing paralytic polio. The injectable form of the polio vaccine (IPV) is incapable of causing paralytic polio and should be used.

    d. The oral preparation of the polio has recently been found to be more favorable and will be used when your son is in need of vaccination.

8. Thirteen-year-old Chandria has been diagnosed with Fifth's disease. She and her caregiver are very upset and ask the nurse how they are going to deal with this situation. Which of the following would be the best response by the nurse?

    a. You will not be able to attend school until the rash on your body is totally gone.

    b. You can expect the rash to recur for weeks with exposure to heat or sun.

    c. This disease is caused by a strain of the herpes virus.

    d. Be sure to drink plenty of fluids, as renal problems commonly occur with this disease.

9. The nurse completes an assessment on a 13-year-old boy. Findings include fever, fatigue, exudative pharyngitis, lymphadenopathy, hepatosplenomegaly, and atypical lymphocytosis. The nurse identifies which of the following as the most likely infectious disease affecting this boy?

    a. diphtheria

    b. pertussis

    c. roseola

    d. infectious mononucleosis

Multiple Response

1. Patrick, a 2-year-old, has puritic lesions caused by an infectious disease. Which of the following will be included by the nurse in teaching the family how to care for Patrick? Select all that apply.

   a. using aspirin to relieve discomfort
   b. using antihistamines such as Benadryl or Atarax
   c. adding baking soda or oatmeal preparations to bath water
   d. keeping fingernails short
   e. placing rubbing alcohol on the lesions
   f. covering all lesions with an air-tight and water-tight dressing

2. A 16-year-old girl sees the nurse in the health clinic and states, "I just found out my boyfriend has gonorrhea. I don't know what to do, or what it even is! I know it is a sex disease, but what am I going to do?" How should the nurse respond? Select all that apply.

   a. You may have it and not even know it because it takes one month before you develop any symptoms.
   b. You will be treated with penicillin G to cure the disease.
   c. Avoid sexual contact until you have taken one day's worth of the antibiotic to avoid spread of the disease.
   d. You should be tested to diagnose presence of the disease, and start treatment to avoid complications such as acute PID, dermatitis, and infertility.
   e. Complications of the disease may include meningitis.
   f. Complications of the disease may include arthritis.

3. Surya, age 15, has been diagnosed with syphilis. She has received education about treatment of the disease. Which of the following statements by Surya would indicate that more teaching is needed?

   a. "I will take the antibiotic until I feel better, then stop it."
   b. "I should use latex condoms to prevent further reinfection."
   c. "I should avoid sexual activity until I am cured."
   d. "If I do not receive treatment for this disease, it could affect my nervous system."
   e. "Once I get over this I will not be able to get syphillis again, just like I had chicken pox and won't get that again."
   f. "I don't have to worry about birth control anymore because now I will not be able to get pregnant."

Critical Thinking/Case Study

The nurse is speaking to a group of parents of newborns. These parents have chosen to take their children to day care facilities when they return to work. The nurse has been asked to address the issue of infectious diseases in day care settings.

1. What questions should the parents ask at the day care center regarding the caregivers who work there?

    _____

    _____

    _____

2. What questions and concerns about sanitation and procedures for handling and preparing food should be asked by the parents?

    _____

    _____

    _____

3. Should the immunization status of other children be of concern to the parents?

    _____

    _____

    _____

4. What questions should the parents ask about the spread and control of illness in the day care center?

    _____

    _____

    _____

5. What are some of the benefits of having the children at the day care center separated by age group and developmental level?

    _____

    _____

    _____

CHAPTER 16

Care of Children Who Are Hospitalized

True or False

1. Until the 19th century, when compared with our views today, children were regarded as small adults, and there was limited recognition of physiologic or psychosocial differences.

   ❏ True   ❏ False

2. Toddlers and preschool children are particularly concerned about intactness of their bodies and feel the distress of exposure and intrusion acutely.

   ❏ True   ❏ False

3. Children in need of radiological examinations are particularly stressed when darkness of the environment is involved.

   ❏ True   ❏ False

4. Caregivers of infants and young children should be encouraged to follow a strict visitation schedule with their hospitalized child, allowing two hours of interaction with the child in the early morning and two hours in the late afternoon to facilitate child transition to the hospital routine.

   ❏ True   ❏ False

5. Most admissions to pediatric units are planned hospitalizations of toddlers under the age of 3.

   ❏ True   ❏ False

6. Prior to preparing a child for surgery, it is helpful to ascertain what the child knows about the surgical procedure and how the child feels.

   ❏ True   ❏ False

7. When working with infants, it is important for the nurse to know that infants at 1 month of age are acutely aware of the absence of their mothers.

   ❑ True ❑ False

8. The basic source of infant satisfaction is through satiation of oral needs.

   ❑ True ❑ False

9. When talking to an 8-year-old about undergoing anesthesia, it would be best for the nurse to tell the child that the child will be "put to sleep" for the procedure.

   ❑ True ❑ False

10. It is very important for school-age children to maintain a sense of industry when hospitalized.

    ❑ True ❑ False

11. Children are not able to experience the therapeutic benefits of guided imagery until 12 years of age.

    ❑ True ❑ False

12. When working with adolescents, nurses should be aware of the fact that the concerns and anxieties of adolescents are often masked by the appearance of sophistication, maturity, and what may be described as bravado.

    ❑ True ❑ False

13. Adolescents who are hospitalized adapt best when they are with younger children so they can assume more of a leadership role on the unit.

    ❑ True ❑ False

14. Fear of the unknown is often the most diffuse and debilitating fear caregivers experience, particularly when children are acutely ill and there is little experience with hospitalization.

    ❑ True ❑ False

15. When children ask questions, it is helpful to respond with short, age-appropriate answers and encourage additional questions.

    ❑ True ❑ False

16. During adolescence, developing a sense of identity is a primary task in development.

    ❑ True ❑ False

Fill in the Blank

1. Philosophical changes have occurred in the care of children from a focus on the disease of children and care of the child to the evolution of _____ centered pediatric care and active participation of _____.

2. _____ was the first nurse to systematically study how children and parents cope with hospitalization and document the effectiveness of nursing in allaying and managing the fears and concerns of hospitalized children.

3. The predominant goal of nursing care for hospitalized children is to preserve their _____ while trying to enhance their _____ in the midst of stress and intrusions into their bodies, their space, and their very being.

4. The primary fears producing stress in hospitalized children are lack of _____, fear of intrusions and _____, and _____ from the significant persons in their lives.

5. _____ is a philosophy of providing therapeutic care through the use of interventions that eliminate or reduce, to the degree possible, the psychological and physical distress experienced by children and families during hospitalization.

6. _____ is an intervention used by nurses where supervised play is the medium used to aid ill and hospitalized children in expressing thoughts and feelings.

7. For a planned admission of a 3-year-old child to the hospital for surgery, the preparation should occur _____ days before the event.

8. When teaching a preschool child about a procedure that is to be performed, the nurse is aware of the fact that preschoolers learn best through _____ and _____ of objects.

9. Recent studies have found that most caregivers want to be _____ when invasive procedures are performed on their children, and nearly all caregivers want to participate in the decision about their presence.

10. When children become ill, injured, or hospitalized, both they and their caregivers feel vulnerable as they seek to maintain some level of _____ and _____ in delicate and difficult situations.

11. Family-centered care is guided by four principles, which are _____, _____, _____, and _____.

12. The three phases of response to separation of young children from their parents due to hospitalization have been described by Robertson as _____, _____, and _____.

Matching

_____ 1. susto

_____ 2. Gladys Sellew

_____ 3. curandera

_____ 4. Eugenia Waechter

a. conducted the first controlled study done directly with children

b. brought richness, reality, community dimension to the field of pediatric nursing

c. traditional healer

d. nervousness and loss of appetite

Multiple Choice

1. The nurse would expect which of the following children and families to experience the highest level of anxiety due to hospitalization?

   a. John, the third child in the family, age 1 week, admitted for phototherapy

   b. Lindsey, age 7, admitted for regulation of blood sugar with transition to an insulin pump

   c. Tom, age 5, who was hit by a car when on his bicycle and who was not wearing a helmet

   d. David, age 13, who has cystic fibrosis and has been admitted to the hospital for a "tune up"

2. Jayne, age 4, is being transported to another area of the hospital for tests by a new nurse. Jayne tells the new nurse she is very afraid because she does not want to get lost. Which of the following responses by the new nurse suggests that intervention by the supervising nurse is indicated?

   a. Don't worry, Jayne, you have a name badge on your wrist and I will take care of you.

   b. Look, Jayne, your room has a brown cat on the front of the door. We will know where to return you after the test.

   c. Let's make a sign to put on your door so we are all sure where to return you.

   d. You will be taken down the hall for the test you need to have done. I'll put this sticker on the door that has your name on it so everyone will know where to take you after the test.

3. Hamilton, age 6, is admitted to the hospital. Which action by an orienting nurse requires intervention by the supervising nurse? The new nurse:

    a. keeps his shoes in sight as a reminder of going home

    b. allows Hamilton to have a space for his own possessions in the hospital room

    c. encourages his parents to bring pictures of his family and friends to the hospital

    d. has Hamilton's family take any transitional objects or favorite things home to avoid the possibility of the items being lost

4. Which age group of children benefits most from group preparation for planned hospitalization?

    a. infants

    b. toddlers

    c. preschoolers

    d. school-age

5. A nurse working on a pediatric unit of a hospital identifies which as most important in the admission process of a child to the unit?

    a. Inform the family of the visiting hours.

    b. Establish a helping, trusting relationship with the child and caregivers.

    c. Ensure that the child will get along with his or her roommate.

    d. Tell the child and caregivers about hospital routines.

6. Saqui is a 4-year-old who is going to have a cast applied to his right leg due to fracture of the femur. What would be the most effective technique to use in preparing Saqui for this procedure?

    a. Show him a video about cast application.

    b. Tell him that it will not be painful and to be a good boy.

    c. Have Saqui use a doll or animal to apply the cast.

    d. Show him a picture of a boy who has a similar type of cast on.

7. Jacob is a 4-year-old who is hospitalized and in need of a bone marrow aspiration sample. The most appropriate place for the nurse to prepare to have this procedure done is:

    a. on Jacob's bed

    b. in the playroom

    c. in the treatment room

    d. in the video room

8. Zed, age 4, is in need of a biopsy of a growth on his right forearm. Considering the developmental needs of preschoolers, the nurse prepares Zed for the procedure with the knowledge that most preschoolers are fearful of intrusive procedures that disrupt the skin integrity because:

   a. They fear their insides may come out.
   b. Scar formation after the procedure is disturbing to them.
   c. Pain during the procedure is feared.
   d. Possibility of an infection is a concern to them.

9. When working with school-age children who are hospitalized, the nurse is aware of the need for school-age children to continue to develop a sense of:

   a. trust
   b. industry
   c. self
   d. autonomy

10. When working with adolescents, it is often difficult for nurses and other health care professionals to establish a helping relationship with them. This is because adolescents:

    a. trust no one
    b. fear intimacy
    c. are seeking independence from parents and those in authority
    d. fear abandonment from their family

11. The role of the nurse in working with caregivers of a hospitalized child is to:

    a. assume total care of the child, allowing the caregivers to rest
    b. make all decisions regarding the needs of the child
    c. provide for all physical and psychosocial needs of the child
    d. help the caregivers to grow during the crisis of illness

Multiple Response

1. When caring for toddlers who are hospitalized, which of the following are appropriate interventions by the nurse? Select all that apply.

   a. Pay attention to efforts by toddlers to feed themselves.
   b. Maintain the same expectations of toilet training that were followed in the home.
   c. Provide opportunities for the toddlers to exercise their will.
   d. Maintain consistency of care and a secure environment for hospitalized toddlers.
   e. Encourage the presence of caregivers.
   f. Expect the toddler to experience separation anxiety.

2. It is time for a hospitalized toddler to take a nap. Which of the following statements by the nurse are appropriate? Select all that apply.

   a. How about getting ready for your nap now?
   b. It is time for your nap now. Would you like to sleep with Cookie Monster or Barney?
   c. Nap time is now. Would you like me to close the door to your room part way or almost all the way?
   d. It is nap time now. Would you like me to read you a story from the red book or the blue book before you go to sleep?
   e. It would make me happy if you took a nap now.
   f. Why don't you be a good kid and take a nap like Joey who is in the room across the hall.

3. When working with school-age children who are hospitalized, which of the following are appropriate methods for the nurse to use when caring for this age group? Select all that apply.

   a. Use humor and jokes to help reduce anxiety.
   b. Use visual aids and stories when teaching the child.
   c. Discourage the child from completing schoolwork until discharge from the hospital.
   d. Encourage contact from friends and introduce other children on the unit who are of similar ages.
   e. Use group preparation for children with similar teaching needs.
   f. Encourage the child to keep a journal.

4. Jethro, age 5, is being discharged from the hospital after an extended stay from a trauma encountered while riding his bike and being hit by a car. Which of the following are appropriate methods for the nurse to use when preparing Jethro and his caregivers for discharge? Select all that apply.

   a. Before discharge from the hospital, encourage Jethro's mother, who has been in his room with him 24 hours a day, to sleep in another room in the hospital for a few nights.

   b. Inform Jethro's caregivers that he will most likely demonstrate regressive behaviors after discharge from the hospital for a period of time.

   c. Expect Jethro to experience more separation anxiety than usual after discharge for a period of time.

   d. Insist that Jethro return to all prehospitalization activities and responsibilities as soon as possible to avoid permanent regressive behavior.

   e. Inform Jethro's caregivers that he will have permanent limitations to his reading comprehension because of the hospital stay.

   f. Inform Jethro's caregivers that all regressive behaviors will return to normal within 48 hours of discharge.

Critical Thinking/Case Study

Compare and contrast the nursing care needs of infants, children, and adolescents as well as their caregivers by various developmental levels.

	Infant	Toddler	Preschool	School-Age	Adolescent
Preparation for hospitalization					
Admission routine					
Nursing interview					
Preparation for surgery					
Preparation for diagnostic/therapeutic procedures					
Nursing care specific to the age group					
Learning method most effective for this age group					
Optimal method of communication					
Interventions to facilitate attainment of developmental tasks specific to this age group					
Effects of separation from caregivers					
Expectations and needs of caregivers specific to the age groups					
Preparation for discharge specific to the age groups					

CHAPTER 17

Chronic Conditions

True or False

1. In the care of children, technology can result in iatrogenic (treatment-induced) chronic conditions.

   ❑ True ❑ False

2. Numerous research studies have concluded that the less visible the condition, the greater the difficulties the child, caregivers, and siblings often have in adjusting to it.

   ❑ True ❑ False

3. While there is some indication that children with chronic conditions, as a group, are at greater risk for maladjustment, results have been inconsistent and have tended to show that most of the children are well adjusted.

   ❑ True ❑ False

4. Several studies have concluded that the severity of the child's condition has a strong relationship to the stability of the parents' marriage.

   ❑ True ❑ False

5. Children with chronic conditions should be encouraged to interact with other children with chronic conditions so they can support one another.

   ❑ True ❑ False

6. Focusing intensely or exclusively on a chronic condition and its trajectory diagnosed in a newborn positively affects bonding.

   ❑ True ❑ False

7. Children with chronic conditions are more likely to be up-to-date with immunizations and basic health screenings than other children due to their frequent interactions with health care professionals.

   ❑ True ❑ False

8. Siblings of children with chronic conditions have no greater risk of developing psychosocial problems that do siblings of healthy children.

   ❑ True   ❑ False

Fill in the Blank

1. _____ refers to a functional limitation that prevents or interferes with a person's ability to perform age-expected activities. A _____ is a barrier imposed by society, the environment, or oneself in response to perceived differences.

2. A situation in which a condition is less visible to others resulting in ambiguity about whether an individual is different from or like others is referred to as _____.

3. _____ is the term used to describe the progression of the chronic condition.

4. The eight adaptive tasks for caregivers of children with chronic conditions are _____, _____, _____, _____, _____, _____, _____, and _____.

5. _____ involves having a person who relieves the usual caregiver of caregiving responsibilities for a period of time.

6. _____ is the tendency for all individuals and cultures to believe their values are the best, the most correct.

Matching

_____ 1. critical-orientation model

a. barrier imposed by society, the environment, or oneself in response to perceived differences

_____ 2. iatrogenic

b. examining the ways physical and social environment stigmatizes and excludes individuals with health issues

_____ 3. handicap

c. condition less visible to others which results in ambiguity about whether the individual is different from or like others

_____ 4. trajectory

_____ 5. marginality

_____ 6. disability

_____ 7. health-orientation model

d. functional limitations that prevent or interfere with a person's ability to perform age-expected activities

e. portrayals of chronic conditions as variations in life

f. treatment-induced chronic conditions

g. progression of the condition

Multiple Choice

1. A nurse who works with children who have chronic conditions practices in a model that facilitates the child's awareness of the changes of the chronic condition as the child progresses through the developmental sequence. In this model, the chronic condition does not assume a central or relevant role in the development of identity or in activities of daily life. Within which model does this nurse practice?

   a. deficit-oriented model
   b. chronic model
   c. health-oriented model
   d. ordinary model

2. The nurse is working with a group of parents whose children have recently been diagnosed with a chronic condition. In teaching this group about adjustment to having a child with a chronic condition, the nurse identifies which of the following as the first stage of the adjustment process?

   a. anger
   b. shock and denial
   c. guilt
   d. acceptance

3. Sue has a 3-year-old son who has just been diagnosed with a chronic condition, and two other children ages 5 and 8. Sue is a single parent who receives little support from the father of her son. Sue states, "What am I going to do about my other two kids? How will this illness affect them and their needs?" The best response for the nurse to make is:

   a. Research suggests that siblings of children with chronic conditions have no greater risk of developing psychosocial problems that do siblings of healthy children.
   b. Families who have a child with a chronic condition are most likely to be dysfunctional.
   c. Children who have a brother or sister with a chronic condition are less likely to care for themselves due to all of the attention given to the sibling with a chronic condition.
   d. Siblings of the child with a chronic condition should assume no responsibility for their care regardless of age or developmental level. This is the responsibility of the caregiver.

4. A 10-year-old child who is permanently in a wheelchair tells the nurse that she feels uncomfortable when people stare at her. The child asks the nurse what she can do about this situation. The best response by the nurse is:

   a. People who stare at you are just showing their ignorance.
   b. You should just pretend that you don't notice them staring.
   c. Ask people who stare at you if they have any questions.
   d. Limit your activities to avoid people who stare at you.

Multiple Response

1. Which of the following statements about school-age children who have chronic conditions are true? Select all that apply.

   a. School-age children may have difficulty understanding why treatments are necessary during symptom-free periods.
   b. School-age children often respond to treatments with manipulative behavior.
   c. School-age children learn best through abstract thought processes.
   d. School-age children may not understand the reason for treatments whose benefits are not immediately apparent.
   e. School-age children are working through trust versus mistrust issues.
   f. School-age children cope best when isolated from others.

2. Which of the following statements about the No Child Left Behind Act of 2002 are true? Select all that apply.

   a. Only children with physical disabilities are affected by this law.
   b. The law increases accountability and flexibility of school systems.
   c. The law requires the use of evidence-based practice.
   d. The law stresses the importance of children performing well in reading and math.
   e. A ratio of one school nurse per 100 students is mandated.
   f. All teachers must have a minimum of a masters degree to start their teaching career.

3. Which of the following are appropriate coping strategies for children with chronic illnesses? Select all that apply.

   a. viewing self as normal
   b. eliciting social support from family
   c. eliciting social support from peers
   d. seeking support from health professionals
   e. denying of condition
   f. not adhering to care regimen

Critical Thinking/Case Study

Lynn, the nurse, is working with the parents of Zachery, age 18 months. Zachery has recently been diagnosed with the chronic condition of muscular dystrophy. In interacting with Zachery and his family, Lynn needs to explore several important dimensions of chronic conditions.

1. What types and kinds of questions should Lynn ask the family concerning the nature and onset of the condition? How does the nurse expect the nature of the onset of the condition to affect the family dynamics?

   _____

   _____

   _____

2. How can Lynn help the family assess and plan for the progression or trajectory of the condition? How will developmental levels Zachery goes through be affected by the condition?

_____

_____

_____

3. What impact, if any, will the condition have on Zachery's appearance? How will the family manage these issues?

_____

_____

_____

4. How can the nurse assess the family's ability to evaluate and plan for effects on the daily functioning of the family due to the condition?

_____

_____

_____

5. What can Lynn do to assist the family in planning how to meet Zachery's physical and psychological needs as he progresses through various developmental levels?

_____

_____

_____

CHAPTER 18

Pain Management

True or False

1. Some health care professionals are still under the impression children do not experience pain or are less sensitive to pain than adults.

   ❑ True   ❑ False

2. Infants do not feel pain.

   ❑ True   ❑ False

3. Infants and children are more sensitive than adults to opioid pain medication.

   ❑ True   ❑ False

4. Children and adolescents will become addicted to opioids that are used to treat pain.

   ❑ True   ❑ False

5. Assessment of pain in toddlers is often difficult because their age-appropriate protest to unpleasant or noxious stimuli may be confused with a response to pain.

   ❑ True   ❑ False

6. Less physical activity than expected is a good indication that a preschooler is experiencing pain.

   ❑ True   ❑ False

7. Use of opioids for pain relief in infants is likely to result in addiction even if the opioids are used for a short period of time.

   ❑ True   ❑ False

8. Opioid analgesics are most effective when administered in large, infrequent doses.

   ❑ True   ❑ False

9. When pain is very severe, opioid analgesics can be titrated to extremely high doses to achieve adequate analgesia with minimal side effects.

   ❏ True   ❏ False

10. Acetaminophen is an example of an anti-inflammatory drug.

    ❏ True   ❏ False

11. Adequate pain control may contribute to a shorter hospital stay, promote quicker return to normal functioning, and lead to a more positive hospital experience.

    ❏ True   ❏ False

12. Sucrose has been found to be an effective analgesic for infants and can be easily delivered through a sucrose-impregnated pacifier.

    ❏ True   ❏ False

Fill in the Blank

1. Pain control using medications or other interventions is called _____.

2. _____ lasts three to five days and is attributed to a specific cause, while _____ lasts for long periods of time or comes and goes frequently over long periods of time.

3. When using the PQRST assessment of pain, the letters represent: P_____, Q_____, R_____, S_____, T_____.

4. _____ are the cornerstone of management for moderate to severe pain.

5. _____ is the gold standard of opioids.

6. _____ is an opioid pain medication for children with the unique side effects of chest wall rigidity with parenteral dosing.

7. The technique of delivering small doses of the pain medication until the desired effect of pain relief is observed is called _____.

8. _____ will reverse respiratory depression of opioid analgesics without reversing the analgesic effects.

9. An individual who has migraines often can predict the onset by an _____ or premonition of their beginning.

Matching

_____ 1. tolerance

_____ 2. addiction

_____ 3. morphine

_____ 4. cutaneous stimulation

_____ 5. FLACC

_____ 6. ceiling dose

a. psychological and physical need to use a medication for a nonprescribed purpose

b. gold standard of opioids

c. point at which there are no longer effects of the medication

d. objective pain scale

e. physical need to increase dose of medication over time to achieve the desired effect

f. application of consistent gentle pressure to the site of pain

Multiple Choice

1. A new nurse is caring for a preschool child who is experiencing pain. Which action by the new nurse requires the supervising nurse to intervene? The new nurse:

   a. identifies less physical activity than expected as an indication the child is in pain

   b. refrains from allowing the child to see or touch any of the equipment that will be used in the procedure to be performed

   c. realizes that a preschool child who is playing may still be in pain

   d. uses drawing or acting out the situation to assist a preschool child in explaining the child's pain

2. Which of the following opioid pain medications is not recommended for children because as the metabolite accumulates, the seizure threshold of the child is lowered?

   a. codeine

   b. fentanyl

   c. methadone

   d. meperidine

3. Which of the following medications is used to reverse respiratory depression of opioid analgesics?

    a. aspirin

    b. Narcan

    c. Valium

    d. hydrocodone

4. Mischiak, age 5, is being discharged to home after sustaining a multiple trauma from a car crash. He has chronic back pain. Which of the following should the nurse encourage Mischiak's caregivers to follow in helping Mischiak cope with his chronic pain?

    a. Ask Mischiak about his pain approximately three times a day to be sure he is feeling all right.

    b. Offer Mischiak secondary gains when he reports having pain to encourage his prompt reporting of the pain experience.

    c. Do not question Mischiak about his perceived experience of pain unless there is a significant change noted.

    d. Schedule household activities around the time when Mischiak is feeling best.

5. When working with school-age children, the nurse is aware of the fact that school-age children:

    a. may assume pain is punishment

    b. act withdrawn when pain is experienced

    c. assume pain will be treated

    d. can conceptualize pain relief

Multiple Response

1. When working with a school-age child who is in pain, the nurse should incorporate which of the following into the plan of care? Select all that apply.

   a. Prepare the child for the procedure to be carried out well in advance of the actual procedure.

   b. Understand the school-age child often views his or her pain as punishment for something he or she caused.

   c. Cover all wounds, as these children often fear their insides will leak out if the skin barrier is not intact.

   d. Break down the procedure into as many steps as possible.

   e. Allow the child to choose which limb a pain medication will be administered in if possible.

   f. Base teaching on the fact that school-age children are abstract thinkers.

2. Yolanda, age 3, was mauled by a neighbor's dog. She is hospitalized and will need to undergo many painful procedures. Which of the following interactions with the family by the nurse in planning for and providing pain relief measures for Yolanda are appropriate? Select all that apply.

   a. Allow Yolanda's caregivers to participate in nonpharmacologic measures to relieve pain such as rubbing, massaging, and holding.

   b. Explore measures Yolanda's caregivers used to relieve her pain in the past.

   c. Understand methods to comfort Yolanda when her caregivers are not available.

   d. Exclusively use pharmacologic measures to relieve Yolanda's pain because of the serious extent of her injuries.

   e. Assess cultural influences related to pain management.

   f. Refrain from use of all opioid analgesics to prevent problems associated with use of these agents in children under the age of 5.

3. When working with infants who are to undergo a painful procedure, the nurse could incorporate which of the following nonpharmacologic pain management techniques in the care of the infant? Select all that apply.

   a. cutaneous stimulation

   b. distraction

   c. guided imagery

   d. use of transcutaneous electrical nerve stimulator (TENS)

   e. hypnosis

   f. progressive muscle relaxation

Critical Thinking/Case Study

Leroy has been practicing nursing on a pediatric unit for the past several years. The unit has recently expanded bed capacity because of trauma services for children that are now being made available at the institution. Leroy has been asked to orient new staff to the pediatric unit. He has been asked to provide specific information to these nurses on pediatric pain assessment and treatment. None of the nurses orienting to the unit have worked with children before. All are experienced medical-surgical nurses who have practiced on adult units.

1. How should Leroy explain pain physiology to the nurses?

    _____

    _____

    _____

2. What would be the most effective method for Leroy to use in summarizing pediatric pain research for these nurses as well as explaining to them about common misconceptions about pediatric pain?

    _____

    _____

    _____

3. Using adult teaching-learning principles, what would be an effective method for Leroy to use in teaching these new nurses the unique pain responses of children in various developmental stages?

    _____

    _____

    _____

4. What are the different pain responses of children in the various developmental stages?

    _____

    _____

    _____

5. How does the pain assessment nurses perform on children differ from that performed on adults?

   _____

   _____

   _____

6. What information should Leroy include in a summary of opioid pain medication for children? How does the dosage differ for adults and children?

   _____

   _____

   _____

7. How does the care of children with chronic pain differ from the care of adults with chronic pain?

   _____

   _____

   _____

CHAPTER 19

Medication Administration

True or False

1. Until recently, children have been excluded from drug trials due to ethical constraints related to informed consent and research risks.

   ❑ True   ❑ False

2. The processes of absorption, distribution, biotransformation, and excretion are the same for neonates, infants, and children, but are different in adults.

   ❑ True   ❑ False

3. There is more rapid absorption of topical medication in infants and children due to greater body surface area to weight ratio.

   ❑ True   ❑ False

4. The immature blood-brain barrier in children under 2 years of age allows relatively easy access to the central nervous system, making these children more sensitive to drugs that act on the brain and increasing the risk of central nervous system toxicity.

   ❑ True   ❑ False

5. The liver is the primary route of drug excretion.

   ❑ True   ❑ False

6. Parents should be removed from the room during medication administration to the infant when at all possible to avoid conflicting feelings the infant has for the parent.

   ❑ True   ❑ False

7. Due to liver immaturity, the drug metabolizing capacity of premature infants and neonates is high.

   ❑ True   ❑ False

8. To administer eye drops or ointment, the child should be placed in a supine position.

   ❑ True   ❑ False

9. To instill otic medication in children under 3 years of age, the pinna should be pulled up and back.

   ❑ True   ❑ False

10. The gastric pH is higher in the newborn and gradually decreases to reach adult level around 2 to 3 years of age.

    ❑ True   ❑ False

Fill in the Blank

1. _____ is concerned with the movement of drugs throughout the body by the processes of absorption, distribution, biotransformation, and excretion.

2. Absorption of drugs administered intramuscularly is _____ and _____ in neonates and infants.

3. _____ is concerned with the biochemical and physiologic effects of drugs and their mechanism of action within the body.

4. Medication administration to pediatric clients adheres to the six rights of _____, _____, _____, _____, _____, and _____.

5. Drugs and their metabolites are excreted from the body in _____, _____, _____, and_____.

6. Drug dosages in children are most commonly calculated on the basis of unit of drug per _____ of body weight or unit of drug per _____.

Matching

_____ 1. bioavailability

_____ 2. absorption

_____ 3. pharmacodynamics

_____ 4. pharmacokinetics

a. process whereby drugs move from the site of administration into the bloodstream

b. movement of drugs through the body

c. drug's concentration and effect once it reaches the site of action

d. portion of drug in the general circulation and availability to exert an effect on the site of action

Multiple Choice

1. The nurse is administering an oral medication to Todd, a 2-year-old boy. The most appropriate action for the nurse to take when administering the medication is:

   a. Follow previously established rituals and routines in medication administration.
   b. Do not allow Todd to touch any of the equipment.
   c. Tell Todd that the medication will be administered now; providing him with a choice would be confusing to a child of this age.
   d. Have Todd's caregivers leave the area when medications are being administered.

2. A new nurse is administering medications to Sasha, a 3-year-old girl. Which action by the new nurse requires the supervising nurse to intervene? The new nurse:

   a. allows Sasha to play with some of the equipment before administering the medication
   b. asks Sasha if she would please take her medication before administering it
   c. does not tell Sasha that she is bad if she does not fully cooperate with the medication administration procedure
   d. asks Sasha if she would like to take her pill with juice or water

3. When preparing to administer an oral medication, it is best for the nurse to:

   a. For infants, administer crushed pills mixed with honey to sweeten the taste.
   b. Place the pill in the posterior of the pharynx to assist a 3-year-old in swallowing.
   c. Not crush enteric-coated tablets.
   d. Mix the medication with essential food or formula to be sure the child receives all of the medication.

4. A nurse has been asked to speak to a group of parents of variously aged children about safe use of medication in the home. Which of the following statements will the nurse include?

   a. Store all medication in a locked place if possible.
   b. Dispose of medications that are no longer needed by burying them in the yard.
   c. Save unused medication to be used at a later time should the same symptoms appear.
   d. Tell children the medication is candy.

5. Which statement by a nurse regarding administration of intravenous medications to a child indicates that more teaching is necessary?

    a. Syringe infusion pumps allow medications to be delivered in a small volume of fluid over a prescribed period of time.

    b. Buitrol administration sets are used for administration of large volumes of fluid, usually 100 mL.

    c. When medications are to be delivered via slow IV push, the port closest to the child should be used.

    d. The SAS or SASH acronym can be used to help the nurse remember the steps of the procedure to administer IV medication through a heparin locked line.

6. When preparing to administer an intramuscular injection to an infant, the nurse is aware of the fact that the preferred injection site for this age group is the:

    a. vastus lateralis

    b. gluteus major

    c. rectus femoris

    d. deltoid

Multiple Response

1. Which of the following are appropriate steps to follow when administering an intramuscular injection to a 3-year old? Select all that apply.

    a. Clean the site with an antiseptic before administration of the medication.

    b. Insert the needle at a 45° angle.

    c. Position the child to relax the muscle being used for the injection.

    d. Have two adults restrain the child when giving the intramuscular injection.

    e. Remove significant others from the environment.

    f. Insert the needle as quickly as safely possible.

2. Which of the following steps are used in the process of administration of nasal medications to infants and young children? Select all that apply.

   a. Use a clean procedure.

   b. Have the child remain in the position used to instill the drops for at least one minute after the medication has been administered.

   c. Position the child with the head hyperflexed.

   d. Restrain the child as needed.

   e. Pinch the child's nose.

   f. Instruct the child to hold his or her breath.

3. Which of the following statements regarding medication administration in the school-age child are true? Select all that apply.

   a. School-age children are immature and should not be active participants in their care.

   b. A reward system may serve as an effective feedback mechanism thus enhancing their cooperation.

   c. School-age children are generally cooperative in taking medication.

   d. School-age children benefit from explanations regarding the purpose of medications.

   e. School-age children are too old for play to be used as an effective teaching method regarding medication administration.

   f. Always tell the school-age child that the medication will taste good so they will take it.

4. When administering oral medications to the pediatric population, the nurse should take which of the following into consideration? Select all that apply.

   a. Shake suspensions before administration to distribute the medication evenly throughout the liquid.

   b. Crush tablets or open capsules and remove the powder or liquid for children under 5 years of age if a liquid form of the medication is not available.

   c. To make the medication more palatable for infants, mix the medication in honey.

   d. Enteric-coated or timed-release tablets should not be crushed.

   e. If a child will not swallow the medication, pinch their nose so they will swallow.

   f. Restraint is never an appropriate intervention as parents may feel their child is being mistreated.

Critical Thinking/Case Study

Wahid is the nurse practicing in a pediatric clinic. On one particular day, Wahid is working with Misha, a student nurse. Misha has identified medication administration in the pediatric population as his primary learning goal for this clinical day.

1. Wahid asks Misha, "So you want to learn more about medication administration in the pediatric population? To be able to do that, you must first understand the general physiologic differences between children and adults in relation to medication administration. What can you tell me about this?" How does Misha reply?

   _____

   _____

   _____

2. Misha has completed a course on growth and development. What developmental considerations will he take into consideration with medication administration to infants, toddlers, preschoolers, school-age children, and adolescents?

   _____

   _____

   _____

3. Wahid asks Misha what he knows about the six rights for medication administration to the pediatric population. How does Misha respond?

   _____

   _____

   _____

4. Misha asks Wahid, "My instructor went over dosage calculations for pediatric medication administration. I'm not sure I really followed. Can you review that with me, please?" What is Wahid's response?

   _____

   _____

   _____

5. Misha and Wahid are working with a family whose son Duane, age 20 months, has been seen by the primary health care provider and has been ordered antibiotics for an ear infection. Duane's mother asks how will she ever be able to give Duane the medication. She states, "Duane is so fussy about what he eats. How will I ever get him to swallow this stuff? Is it okay if I just give him the medicine until he feels better?" Provide Misha and Wahid's response.

    _____

    _____

    _____

6. Wahid picks up the next chart and sees that the next clients to be seen are a family of three children ages 3 months, 2 years, and 9 years. All require intramuscular medication administration to be kept up-to-date with immunizations. Wahid asks Misha, "What are the injection sites we can use for each child? Which needle length and gauge should we use for each child? What can we do to plan for safe medication administration for each child? Should we let the mother stay in the room?" What does Misha say?

    _____

    _____

    _____

CHAPTER 20

Loss and Bereavement

True or False

1. Children experience loss and bereavement through a myriad of situations such as relocation, loss of possessions, pet loss, and parental separation/divorce as well as death of a person.

   ❏ True   ❏ False

2. Because children view pets as friends, the loss of a pet through death (or through the pet's running away or being stolen) may be the child's first real experience with loss, separation, and grieving.

   ❏ True   ❏ False

3. Children of divorce are no more likely to have academic problems, exhibition of externalized behaviors and internalized disorders, lower self-esteem, and problems in their relationships with parents, siblings, and peers when compared to children whose parents have not divorced.

   ❏ True   ❏ False

4. Adolescents are capable of understanding and conceptualizing death as permanent and universal, but there is often an exclusion of the self from this concept; in other words, "It won't happen to me."

   ❏ True   ❏ False

5. Children may have long periods when they are overcome with grief, followed by an interval when they do not seem to be affected by the loss.

   ❏ True   ❏ False

6. Few events hold as much potential to disrupt a child's family pattern of life and place the child at risk for enduring psychological stress than the death of a parent.

   ❏ True   ❏ False

7. Following the death of a child, surviving siblings are often overlooked as support is generally provided to the grieving parent.

   ❑ True   ❑ False

8. Because sibling relationships run the gamut of emotions, a surviving sibling may experience not only sorrow at the loss of a brother or sister, but also guilt about something that was thought or said about the deceased.

   ❑ True   ❑ False

9. The literature on children's understanding of death reveals that on average, children under the age of 4 have little to no understanding of the concept of death.

   ❑ True   ❑ False

10. The decision to perform an autopsy on a child is a requirement of law when death is caused by unnatural causes such as murder or suicide, when it occurs within 24 hours of hospitalization, or if death occurs at home or in an institution when a person has not been under the care of a physician.

    ❑ True   ❑ False

Fill in the Blank

1. Two major factors in children's reaction to loss are _____ and _____.

2. _____ is the assumption of the caregiver (parental) role.

3. The concept of death can be defined as having four distinct components: _____, _____, _____, and _____.

4. _____ is an individual's response to loss and is viewed as a natural and healthy process, _____ is seen as an adaptation to loss, and _____ is the process one goes through on his or her way to adaptation.

5. Kübler-Ross identified the five distinct stages of the grieving process as _____, _____, _____, _____, and _____.

6. Worden's four tasks of mourning are _____, _____, _____, and _____.

Matching

_____ 1. causality

_____ 2. bereavement

_____ 3. grief

_____ 4. depression

_____ 5. universality

a. adaptation to stress

b. death is inevitable

c. individual response to loss

d. death has internal and external causes

e. reality of situation subconsciously beginning to take hold

Multiple Choice

1. The nurse is working with an 8-year-old child named Bobby whose parents have recently divorced. The parents ask the nurse, "We don't know what is wrong with him. We have given Bobby all he has asked for because we know this is a difficult time for him. Why is he being so difficult?" The best response by the nurse is:

    a. I'm not sure. Have you tried counseling?

    b. You must have done something to make him feel so bad; usually 8-year-olds are easily adaptable to change.

    c. Children in this age group may have fantasies of reunification of parents and family and may lie in an attempt to make this fantasy come true.

    d. You probably have low self-esteem because of the divorce. Are you sure the problem is not yours?

2. According to Piaget, a 16-year-old's understanding of death can be described as:

    a. causality

    b. selective universality (does not include self)

    c. avoidable

    d. reversible and temporary

3. The nurse is working with Max, a 7-year-old whose father was tragically killed in a motor vehicle crash. Max tells the nurse, "I was so bad. My daddy left for work, and he never came back. I promise to be a good boy. I want my daddy to come back; I miss him. I'll be a good boy now." Max is in which phase of the grieving process according to Kübler-Ross?

    a. acceptance

    b. denial

    c. anger

    d. bargaining

4. Tia is 14 and graduating from junior high to high school. Her mother died last year from breast cancer. Tia lives with her grandmother and father. A graduation ceremony and party are planned for the class. Tia's teacher asks the school nurse to see Tia because she has not been herself. Tia does not want to get involved with the planning of the ceremony or party, and this is very unlike her. Tia has also been unkind to several of her classmates when discussion of parental roles in the ceremony occurred. The school nurse assesses Tia as most likely being in which phase of Worden's tasks of mourning?

    a. Task I
    b. Task II
    c. Task III
    d. Task IV

5. The most appropriate intervention for the school nurse to take when working with an adolescent who experienced the death of a parent to continue with everyday life activities is to:

    a. Explain death in age-appropriate terms.
    b. Help the teenager to determine the relationship the parent had in his or her life.
    c. Help the teenager to find a place for her parent in his or her heart.
    d. Acknowledge the teenager's feelings or behaviors associated with the loss.

6. The most common psychosocial response by the adolescent as a reaction to loss, whether it be due to separation or death, is:

    a. distancing self from parents and family
    b. fantasies of parental reunification
    c. fear of being rejected
    d. anxiety

7. To assist the family in adjusting to the loss of a newborn, it is most important for the nurse to:

    a. Present the baby to the parents just as would be done if the newborn were alive.
    b. Cover the newborn's face.
    c. Allow the parents to stay with the baby for about five to ten minutes and then encourage them to leave.
    d. Do not allow the parents to hold the newborn.

8. Mia is a 6-year-old girl with a metastatic brain tumor. Her parents are extremely upset. They have not told Mia anything about the disease process. The parents say to the nurse, "We're so afraid. We feel so bad. What are we going to do? The doctors say she may not have much longer to live." The nurse identifies the parents as most likely being in which phase of familial experience of life-threatening illness?

   a. chronic phase

   b. recovery phase

   c. terminal phase

   d. diagnostic/acute phase

9. After experiencing the death of his 3-year-old child from leukemia, the father asks the nurse if his child will have to have an autopsy. The child was in the hospital for two weeks before he died. "He has been through so much, does that autopsy have to be done?" The best response by the nurse is:

   a. Yes, it is hospital policy that all children under 5 have an autopsy regardless of parental request.

   b. You really want to know what caused the death of your son, don't you? An autopsy is the only way to find out exactly what the cause of death was.

   c. Yes, it was not an accident, so we have to find out what killed him.

   d. Most likely not. Your son was in the hospital for more than 24 hours, he was under the care of a physician, and the death was a result of leukemia.

Multiple Response

1. The nurse is working with a group of junior high students who survived a bus accident. A drunk driver hit the bus of the soccer team. Both spectators and players were on the bus. Three of the students were killed along with the bus driver. When working with the survivors and students in the school, the nurse understands that which of the following are true? Select all that apply.

   a. Students who were not on the bus may suffer the effects of the disaster.
   b. Counseling should be provided for the students for one week in school, and after this time, counseling should occur out of the school setting on the students' own time.
   c. Acknowledge this was a crime against the community and not just individuals.
   d. Expect only the students who were on the bus to experience rage, sleep disturbances, repeated thoughts about the incident, increased alertness to danger, and fear of attending any events with an environment similar to the traumatic incident.
   e. All school activities related to sports should be cancelled for at least six weeks.
   f. Any school activity unrelated to sports should be cancelled for at least four weeks.

2. When working with children who have experienced long-term traumatic events such as the effects of natural disasters, the nurse expects the children to experience which of the following? Select all that apply.

   a. emotional maturation
   b. depression
   c. disrupted moral development
   d. masked emotions
   e. sleep disturbances
   f. anxiety

3. When working with a group of parents who have questions about the effect of divorce on children, which of the following statements will the nurse include? Select all that apply.

   a. The age of the child at the time of the divorce has significant impact on their response to the situation.
   b. Preschool children experience fear of abandonment.
   c. Adolescent children fantasize about methods to get their parents back together.
   d. School-age children internalize their sadness and withdraw.
   e. Adolescents often sever personal relationships when parents divorce.
   f. Toddlers often feel that they are being punished for doing something wrong.

Critical Thinking/Case Study

The nurse is providing care to a terminally ill 8-year-old child named Sam and his family in the home. Sam is the middle child. He has an older sister Mera, age 10, and a baby sister Savanah, age 2. Sam's parents are divorced. His father has remarried. He and his new wife are expecting their first child any day. Sam's mother works full-time and is in school part-time to complete her college degree. The parents have joint custody of Sam and the girls. The children live with mom during the week and they go to their dad's home on the weekends. This is a very stressful time for everyone.

1. What are the nurse's primary goals in the care of Sam?

   _____

   _____

   _____

2. What are the nurse's primary goals in the care of Sam's family?

   _____

   _____

   _____

3. What does the nurse need to analyze about herself before she is able to care for Sam and his family?

   _____

   _____

   _____

4. Sam's older sister asks the nurse why she cannot just help her brother get better. How can the nurse best respond?

   _____

   _____

   _____

5. Sam's mother asks the nurse, "I don't know what I am going to do. Sam's father is more concerned about his new baby than he is about his own dying son. I don't ever get a break from the kids. I feel so guilty because I don't know how much more time I have with Sam. I am so tired." What might the nurse suggest?

_____

_____

_____

6. Despite trying every known treatment for Sam, he is not responding to any of them. His death is imminent. The nurse thinks that she is really feeling burned out, that she just cannot go to that house anymore and see this young child die. What should the nurse do to take care of herself?

_____

_____

_____

CHAPTER 21

Fluid and Electrolyte Alterations

True or False

1. Changes in diet and activity habits have lead to an increase in average body fat content, which has contributed to overestimation of total body water estimates of infants and children from previous decades.

   ❑ True   ❑ False

2. Infants and young children have a higher basal metabolic rate than adults.

   ❑ True   ❑ False

3. Respiratory alkalosis occurs when the carbon dioxide level is too high.

   ❑ True   ❑ False

4. Metabolic acidosis in children most frequently results from diarrhea and diabetic ketoacidosis.

   ❑ True   ❑ False

5. The most reliable method for diagnosing dehydration is measurement of acute weight loss.

   ❑ True   ❑ False

6. Prevention of skin breakdown is paramount in the treatment of children with edema.

   ❑ True   ❑ False

7. Salmonella is a virus that frequently is the cause of acute gastroenteritis.

   ❑ True   ❑ False

8. Breast milk, cow's milk, and full-strength formula should be avoided when the child has acute gastroenteritis.

   ❑ True   ❑ False

9. The most effective treatment for gastroenteritis is prevention, specifically good handwashing.

   ❑ True   ❑ False

10. The priority treatment for major burns is respiratory management.

    ❑ True   ❑ False

11. Intravenous morphine sulfate is contraindicated in the treatment of children with major burns.

    ❑ True   ❑ False

12. Play therapy is used to help the child with burns deal with the frustrations of burn therapy.

    ❑ True   ❑ False

13. Glucose must be present in order for the intestines to absorb sodium chloride.

    ❑ True   ❑ False

14. Diarrhea is the second leading cause of death in children in the world.

    ❑ True   ❑ False

15. Rotovirus can live on toys and clothing for several days.

    ❑ True   ❑ False

Fill in the Blank

1. Four key physiologic factors are responsible for the fluid and electrolyte differences between children and adults. These include: _____, _____, _____, and _____.

2. Some examples of hypertonic intravenous fluids include: _____, _____, and _____.

3. Sodium, the major extracellular electrolyte, is responsible for establishing and maintaining _____ (the concentration of solute within a solution measured by the number of moles per liter of water) and volume of extracellular fluid.

4. An elevated serum potassium level can cause _____ irritability that can lead to _____.

5. _____ is indicated by a blood pH below 7.35, while _____ is indicated by a blood pH above 7.45.

6. The three types of dehydration are _____, _____, and _____.

7. _____ is defined as diarrheal disease of rapid onset with or without accompanying manifestations such as nausea, vomiting, fever, and abdominal pain.

8. The traditional BRAT diet consists of _____, _____, _____, and _____.

9. The four major types of burns are _____, _____, _____, and _____.

10. The thick leatherlike dead skin often seen after burn injury is called _____.

11. _____ is an incision made into constricting burned skin to restore peripheral blood circulation.

12. _____ is the removal of dead tissue from the burn site and is associated with severe pain.

13. Skin grafts from cadaver skin are called _____, while skin grafts from pigs are called _____.

14. The skin for a(n) _____ is taken from an unburned area of the child's own skin.

Matching

_____ 1. Norwalk

_____ 2. solute

_____ 3. salmonella

_____ 4. hypovolemia

_____ 5. acidosis

_____ 6. Ringers lactate

_____ 7. alkalosis

_____ 8. Dextrose 5% in 0.45 normal saline

_____ 9. hydrostatic pressure

_____ 10. water

_____ 11. oncotic presure

_____ 12. dehydration

_____ 13. Giardia lambia

a. substance dissolved in a solution

b. bacteria

c. virus

d. hypertonic solution

e. blood pH less that 7.35

f. isotonic solution

g. decrease circulating blood volume

h. hypotonic solution

i. deficit of total body water

j. amount of plasma protein present in vascular system also responsible for holding fluids in capillaries

k. blood pH greater than 7.45

l. parasite

m. pressure or blood against capillary wall generated when the heart contracts

Multiple Choice

1. Which of the following statements about hyponatremia is true?

   a. Cardiac irregularity is the earliest clinical manifestation.

   b. It is often found as a result of diarrhea and vomiting.

   c. An early symptom is muscle spasms.

   d. A serum sodium level of 148 mEq/L is expected.

2. Which of the following statements is true regarding potassium?

   a. The normal serum potassium range for a child is 5.5–6.5 mEq/L.

   b. Any imbalance will greatly affect neurologic function.

   c. High and low levels of potassium are most easily recognized through electrocardiographic changes of the P wave.

   d. Renal failure often results in hyperkalemia.

3. Which of the following clinical conditions is associated with respiratory alkalosis?

   a. muscular dystrophy

   b. anxiety

   c. diabetes mellitus

   d. drug overdose

4. Which of the following is the appropriate management approach for the nurse to take when working with a child who has respiratory alkalosis?

   a. Administer sodium bicarbonate.

   b. Encourage slow ventilation.

   c. Administer oxygen.

   d. Administer potassium chloride.

5. A burn that involves the epidermis and dermis and extends into the subcutaneous tissue would most likely be referred to as which type of burn?

   a. superficial

   b. partial thickness

   c. full thickness

   d. second degree

6. Kim, age 8, has sustained a major thermal burn. After establishment of airway patency and breathing, the priority nursing consideration is:

   a. wound care

   b. adequate fluid replacement

   c. assessment for signs of infection

   d. monitoring intake of calories

Multiple Response

1. When administering potassium chloride intravenously to a child, the nurse will take which of the following actions? Select all that apply.

   a. Be sure the child is able to void 1–2 mL/kg/hr before adding potassium to the IV.
   b. Administer the potassium IV push at a rate of 1 mL per minute.
   c. When adding potassium to an IV bag, shake it to make sure the potassium is equally distributed.
   d. Never give more than 40 mEq/L at a rate not to exceed 1 mEq/kg/hr.
   e. Hold all potassium supplementation for a serum level of 3.0 mEq/L.
   f. Assess the child for change in level of consciousness as the first indication of potassium imbalance.

2. Which of the following statements about children and edema are true? Select all that apply.

   a. Edema is associated with renal failure.
   b. Most diuretics cause potassium losses.
   c. Positioning an edematous limb below the level of the heart will facilitate reabsorption of extracellular fluid.
   d. Edema is often noted in the periorbital area of the child.
   e. Meticulous skin care is needed for the child who has edema.
   f. Potassium plays a major role in the regulation of water balance in the body.

3. Which of the following clinical conditions is associated with hyperkalemia? Select all that apply.

   a. administration of intravenous regular insulin
   b. renal failure
   c. hemolysis
   d. tissue necrosis
   e. burn injury
   f. crush injuries

Critical Thinking/Case Study

Moira, age 8, has sustained a scald injury over 12% of her body. Moira spilled a pot of boiling water on her upper trunk when she tried to help her mother with dinner preparations. She has an inhalation injury from the steam and is in an extreme amount of pain.

1. Why is Moira more susceptible to fluid and electrolyte imbalances when compared to an adult?

   _____

   _____

   _____

2. What are the priority nursing interventions in the treatment of Moira?

   _____

   _____

   _____

3. Which electrolyte imbalances does the nurse suspect Moira as being at high risk for due to her injury? What are common signs and symptoms of them? What are the expected treatments for these imbalances?

   _____

   _____

   _____

4. How will the nurse plan to care for Moira, who has now developed respiratory acidosis?

   _____

   _____

   _____

5. Outline the assessment techniques the nurse will use to determine Moira's fluid status.

   _____

   _____

   _____

6. Review the expected treatment of Moira in relation to response of the cardiovascular, renal, central nervous, and metabolic systems due to the major burn injury.

    _____

    _____

    _____

7. Moira weighs 28 kilograms. Using the Parkland formula, calculate her fluid replacement needs for the first 24 hours.

    _____

    _____

    _____

8. Moira is in extreme pain. Plan a management program for her pain.

    _____

    _____

    _____

9. Skin grafts are applied to Moira's upper trunk. Develop a plan of care to promote healing of the graft site and donor site.

    _____

    _____

    _____

10. Because the burn injury occurred at home when Moira's mother was also caring for her younger brother, the mother has much guilt and anxiety. How can the nurse assist the family in dealing with the psychological implications of the burn injury?

    _____

    _____

    _____

CHAPTER 22

Genitourinary Alterations

True or False

1. By school-age, the kidneys are of mature size and weight.

    ❑ True   ❑ False

2. Children are more susceptible to renal trauma from compression force to the abdomen when compared to adults.

    ❑ True   ❑ False

3. Cystitis is an example of an upper urinary tract infection.

    ❑ True   ❑ False

4. Boys who are uncircumcised are as likely to have urinary tract infections as those who are circumcised.

    ❑ True   ❑ False

5. Enuresis differs from incontinence in that incontinence results from a structural abnormality, usually an anatomic malformation.

    ❑ True   ❑ False

6. Overdoses of imipramine cause cardiac arrhythmias.

    ❑ True   ❑ False

7. Surgery for a child with hypospadias is usually performed before the child is 8 months of age.

    ❑ True   ❑ False

8. Common complications of anticholinergics used to alleviate bladder spasm include facial flushing and dry mouth.

    ❑ True   ❑ False

9. Inguinal hernias are usually painless.

    ❑ True   ❑ False

10. The mainstay of treatment for nephrotic syndrome is corticosteroid therapy.

    ❑ True   ❑ False

11. Most renal transplants are lost to rejection.

    ❑ True   ❑ False

12. Continuous renal replacement therapy (CRRT) is used in clients who have difficulty in handling large fluid and electrolyte shifts.

    ❑ True   ❑ False

13. Vesicoureteral reflux (VUR) is the most common anatomic disorder affecting the genito-urinary tract.

    ❑ True   ❑ False

Fill in the Blank

1. Infection of the bladder is called _____, while infection of the kidney is referred to as _____.

2. _____ is a rare, serious congenital anomaly of the abdominal wall and underlying structure failing to fuse, producing exposed bladder and urethra, pubic bone separation, and associated genital and anal abnormalities.

3. White blood cells found in the urine are called _____.

4. Involuntary voiding of urine beyond the expected age at which voluntary control should be achieved is called _____.

5. Some treatments that can be used separately or in combination to treat children with wetting problems include _____, _____, _____, and _____.

6. When a child has bed-wetting problems, foods and beverages to eliminate include _____, _____, _____, _____, _____, and _____.

7. _____ is defined as the backflow of urine from the bladder up the ureter to the kidney.

8. _____ is a common congenital malformation in which the urethral meatus is on the ventral surface (underside) of the penis.

9. Associated conditions that may occur with hypospadias include _____ (downward curvature of the penis and an incomplete foreskin), _____, and _____.

10. Failure of one or both of the testes to descend through the inguinal canal into the scrotum is called _____ or _____.

11. A(n) _____ is a scrotal or inguinal swelling, or both, that includes the abdominal contents, while a(n) _____ is a collection of peritoneal fluid in the scrotal sac.

12. Before surgery to correct an inguinal hernia, the nurse is responsible to assess for complications such as _____ or strangulation of a portion of the bowel leading to circulation impairment and tissue necrosis.

13. Nephrotic syndrome is a clinical entity characterized by massive _____ and _____ leading to _____ and _____.

14. The clinical manifestations of hemolytic uremic syndrome are a triad of symptoms that include _____, _____, and _____.

Matching

_____ 1. cryptorchordism

_____ 2. trigone

_____ 3. oxybutynin chloride

_____ 4. incontinence

_____ 5. pyuria

_____ 6. hydrocele

_____ 7. dysuria

_____ 8. chordee

_____ 9. hypospadias

_____ 10. imipramine hydrochloride

_____ 11. diurnal enuresis

_____ 12. prepuce

a. involuntary loss of urine at daytime

b. difficult or painful urination

c. Ditropan

d. undescended testes

e. anatomic malformation involving loss of urine

f. collection of peritoneal fluid in the scrotal sac

g. Tofranil

h. white blood cells in the urine

i. urethral meatus located on the ventral surface of the penis

j. triangular area at the base of the bladder

k. downward curvature of the penis and incomplete foreskin

l. skin over the glans penis

Multiple Choice

1. Evona is a 7-year-old girl who has had multiple urinary tract infections. Which statement by her mother indicates that more teaching is necessary?

    a. I will have Evona increase the amount of water she usually drinks.
    b. I will encourage Evona to void frequently and completely.
    c. When Evona starts to obtain relief from the infection, I will stop antibiotic therapy to avoid developing resistance to the medication.
    d. I will teach Evona to wipe from front to back for personal hygiene.

2. Which of the following medication orders will the nurse question for the treatment of enuresis?

    a. furosemide (Lasix)
    b. imipramine hydrochloride (Tofranil)
    c. desmopressin (DDAVP)
    d. oxybutynin chloride (Ditropan)

3. Shamal is a 10-year-old boy who has been placed on desmopressin acetate (DDAVP) by his primary care provider to treat enuresis. When teaching Shamal and his family about adverse reactions to his medications, which one of the following statements is included by the nurse?

    a. Nosebleeds are a possible adverse reaction of this medication.
    b. Shamal will most likely have changes in his personality.
    c. Be very careful on hot days, as Shamal will most likely experience heat intolerance.
    d. Be sure Shamal eats plenty of roughage, as constipation is a common complication associated with this medication.

4. Carlos is an infant who has been diagnosed with cryptorchidism. His father asks the nurse, "If surgery needs to be performed on my son, when will it most likely occur?" The best response by the nurse is:

    a. before 1 year of age
    b. between 1 and 2 years of age
    c. between 3 and 4 years of age
    d. between 5 and 6 years of age

5. Xavier is a 1-month-old baby boy who has been diagnosed with cryptorchidism. He has been placed on human chorionic gonadotropin (HCG). Which statement by his mother indicates more teaching is indicated?

    a. I can expect increased growth of Xavier's penis.
    b. Xavier will most likely have the development of pubic hair.
    c. HCG is used to promote descent of the testis.
    d. Pubic hair will persist after the HCG is stopped.

6. Theo is an 11-year-old boy who has been admitted to the hospital with acute glomerulo-nephritis. Which action by the new nurse requires the supervising nurse to intervene? The new nurse:

    a. administers diuretics as ordered
    b. observes for signs of edema
    c. provides a high-protein diet
    d. places a pillow under edematous extremities

Multiple Response

1. Latisha, age 13, is being discharged to home after hospitalization for acute glomerulo-nephritis following a strep throat infection. Which of the following statements should be made to Latisha and her caregivers? Select all that apply.

    a. Elevate your lower extremities when sitting in a chair.
    b. Drink as much diet pop as you like; you need the fluids, and it does not have sugar.
    c. Call your primary care provider if you experience changes in your breathing ability.
    d. Inform the primary care provider if you becomes restless.
    e. Eat foods that are high in potassium such as bananas because your potassium level most often falls low with this condition.
    f. Eat foods that are high in salt because you need to retain fluid.

2. Rob, age 14, has chronic renal failure. He and his caregivers have not been compliant with his care regimen. The nurse provides Rob and his caregivers with an overview of common components of the care of an individual in chronic renal failure. Which of the following statements will the nurse include? Select all that apply.

   a. Maintain high phosphorus levels to ensure skeletal development.
   b. Restrict protein intake.
   c. Provide vitamin D supplementation as ordered to maintain calcium levels.
   d. Take aluminum-based antacids as needed.
   e. Weigh yourself daily.
   f. Drink fluids until your urine is a pale color.

3. Which of the following statements about peritoneal dialysis in children is/are true? Select all that apply.

   a. It requires the placement of a catheter into the peritoneal cavity.
   b. Peritoneal dialysis may take place in the home.
   c. It is the treatment of choice for infants requiring dialysis because of the rapid removal of fluids and waste.
   d. Peritoneal dialysis usually does not require a heparinized line.
   e. Infections rarely occur.
   f. Caregivers can be taught to perform this procedure.

4. Which of the following statements about continuous renal replacement therapy (CRRT) are true? Select all that apply.

   a. Clients receiving CRRT have fewer episodes of hemodynamic instability and disequilibrium syndrome.
   b. If two veins are used for continuous venovenous hemofiltration (CVVH), a pump is required to move the blood throughout the circuitry system.
   c. CRRT is a form of hemofiltration.
   d. Specially trained hemodialysis nurses are needed to care for the child receiving CRRT.
   e. CRRT is easily performed in the home.
   f. The peritoneum is the membrane providing the space for diffusion of fluids.

Critical Thinking/Case Study

Tia is an 11-year-old girl who is in end-stage renal disease. She is on a list awaiting renal transplantation. Her caregivers are very confused and frightened. Tia's father asks the nurse how this could have happened to his little girl. The nurse has been Tia's case manager since the events leading to this situation began. Tia's father is ready and desires to learn more about how Tia has diminished to the point of needing a kidney transplant.

1. Tia's father asks how this all began. The nurse informs him that Tia had a group A beta hemolytic streptococcal infection that led to the development of acute glomerulonephritis. How should the nurse describe this progression from throat infection to renal disease?

   _____

   _____

   _____

2. In the course of treatment, Tia was progressing well when she developed nephrotic syndrome. How should the nurse explain to Tia's father how this could have occurred and its effect on Tia's kidneys?

   _____

   _____

   _____

3. Tia did well for about nine months, then she fell off a trampoline and sustained a pelvic fracture. Due to blood loss, Tia required a blood transfusion. Tia was given the wrong blood and had a blood transfusion reaction and went into acute renal failure. How should the nurse explain how a blood transfusion reaction can affect an individual's kidneys?

   _____

   _____

   _____

4. Tia did not recover from the acute renal failure and was placed on peritoneal dialysis. Her father asks the nurse to review how that worked. What would be an appropriate way to explain peritoneal dialysis?

   _____

   _____

   _____

5. Tia was then placed on hemodialysis. The father wishes to learn more about how hemodialysis was used to supplement his daughter's failing kidneys. What information should the nurse give Tia's father?

_____

_____

_____

6. Now that dialysis is no longer effective in maintaining Tia's homeostasis, she is on a list for kidney transplantation. Her father would like to know what type of care Tia will need if and when she receives a kidney. How should the nurse respond?

_____

_____

_____

CHAPTER 23

Gastrointestinal Alterations

True or False

1. Peristalsis is greater in the older child than in the infant.

    ❑ True   ❑ False

2. Clefts of the hard or soft palate are surgically closed at approximately 1 year of age.

    ❑ True   ❑ False

3. Long-term consequences of cleft lip and palate may include speech difficulties, malocclusion problems, and hearing problems.

    ❑ True   ❑ False

4. In esophageal atresia, initial treatment is aimed at preventing aspiration pneumonia until surgical repair of the defect is completed.

    ❑ True   ❑ False

5. Blood in the stool provides a definite diagnosis of Hirschsprung's disease.

    ❑ True   ❑ False

6. Infants with gastroesophageal reflux should be placed in an infant seat as a mode of treatment.

    ❑ True   ❑ False

7. Nursing management of children with celiac disease includes adherence to a gluten-free diet until late adolescence followed by progression to a normal diet.

    ❑ True   ❑ False

8. Biliary atresia is the single most frequent indicator for liver transplantation in children.

    ❑ True   ❑ False

9. Umbilical hernias are found most commonly in African-American low birth-weight females.

    ❑ True   ❑ False

10. Meckel's diverticulum is the most common congenital malformation of the gastrointestinal tract.

    ❑ True   ❑ False

11. The American Academy of Pediatrics (AAP) recommends that syrup of ipecac to induce vomiting no longer be used routinely as poison treatment in the home and that clinicians advise caregivers to discard any ipecac they have in the house.

    ❑ True   ❑ False

12. Cholestasis is interruption of bile flow.

    ❑ True   ❑ False

Fill in the Blank

1. Infants require small frequent feedings because of _____ stomach capacity, _____ peristalsis, and _____ stomach emptying rate.

2. Infants are deficient in several digestive enzymes that are usually not sufficient until 4 to 6 months of age. They include _____, responsible for initial digestion of carbohydrates, and _____, responsible for hydrolyzing lactose.

3. When an infant has hypertrophic pyloric stenosis, a surgical procedure called a _____ is the treatment of choice in which the circular muscle fibers are released, opening the passage from the stomach into the duodenum.

4. The treatment for a child with a cleft lip and palate is complex and involves many members of the health care team, including: _____, _____, _____, _____, _____, _____, _____, and _____.

5. Feeding is an important nursing concern for the baby with a cleft lip or palate. One readily available method is the use of a standard nipple and bottle with the ESSR method: E_____, S_____, S_____, and R_____.

6. _____ is characterized by incomplete formation of the esophagus so it terminates before reaching the stomach.

7. The acronym VACTERL has been used to describe the condition of multiple anomalies in infants with tracheoesophageal defects: V_____, A_____, C_____, T_____, E_____, R_____, L_____.

8. The nurse recognizes the four signs and symptoms that classically describe an infant with intussusception as: _____, _____, _____, and _____.

9. The family of an infant with intussusception tells the nurse, "The doctor told us they are going to blow air into the intestine of our baby to try to relieve the problem. What is the name of this procedure?" The nurse replies: _____.

10. Complete the following mnemonic for peritonitis: P_____, E_____, R_____, I_____, T_____, O_____, N_____, I_____, T_____, I_____, S_____.

11. When teaching families, the nurse informs them that hepatitis _____ causes acute hepatitis, whereas hepatitis _____ and _____ cause chronic infections.

12. _____ occurs when one segment of the bowel telescopes into the lumen of an adjacent segment of intestine.

13. _____ is the most common intra-abdominal condition requiring surgery during the neonatal period.

Matching

_____ 1. steatorrhea

_____ 2. Hirschsprung's disease

_____ 3. gastroschisis

_____ 4. meconium

_____ 5. anastomosis

_____ 6. ulcerative colitis

_____ 7. intussusception

_____ 8. dysphagia

_____ 9. melena

_____ 10. celiac disease

a. first feces of the newborn

b. surgical connection of two tubular structures

c. one segment of the bowel telescopes into the lumen of an adjacent segment of the intestine

d. large amounts of unabsorbed fats excreted in the stool

e. difficulty swallowing

f. gluten-sensitive enteropathy

g. black, tarry stool

h. congenital defect in the abdominal wall

i. inflammation of the mucosa and submucosa of the colon and rectum

j. motility disorder caused by the absence of parasympathetic ganglionic cells in the large intestine

Multiple Choice

1. When teaching the caregivers of an infant with hypertrophic pyloric stenosis (HPS), which of the following statements will the nurse include?

   a. The condition usually presents when the infant is 3 to 4 weeks of age.
   b. When the baby vomits it will be green.
   c. The infant usually has large bowel movements.
   d. The infant is hungry in spite of vomiting and will want to feed again.

2. The priority nursing focus of care in the preoperative period for the infant with hypertrophic pyloric stenosis focuses on:

   a. preoperative teaching
   b. pain management
   c. developmental assessment
   d. rehydration and correction of the electrolyte imbalance

3. When working with the family of a baby with a craniofacial anomaly, the nurse recognizes that the initial reaction by the family is usually:

   a. grief
   b. feelings of isolation
   c. shock
   d. feelings of failure or inadequacy

4. The nurse working with a baby immediately after surgery for cleft lip repair places major emphasis on:

   a. pain relief
   b. family education
   c. protection of the operative area
   d. mobility exercises for the baby

5. The maternal history of a baby with a gastrointestinal obstruction would most likely include which of the following?

   a. gestational diabetes
   b. polyhydramnios
   c. hypertension
   d. fluid retention

6. The nurse is assessing Kunal, a 12-year-old who has abdominal discomfort. After obtaining a history from Kunal and his family and performing a physical examination on Kunal, the nurse has collected the following information. Kunal was fine until eight hours ago when he complained of his "belly hurting." Four hours ago the pain was at his belly button area and now is located in his right lower abdomen. He now does not feel right, does not want to eat, and feels like he could vomit. After gathering this information, what does the nurse suspect Kunal of having?

   a. gastroenteritis
   b. appendicitis
   c. colitis
   d. food poisoning

7. Lisa, age 13, has been diagnosed with inflammatory bowel disease. At this point, it is not known whether she has Crohn's disease or ulcerative colitis. Lisa asks the nurse to explain the difference. In comparing Crohn's disease to ulcerative colitis, the nurse would tell Lisa that ulcerative colitis:

   a. involves more blood in the stool
   b. affects the entire GI tract
   c. involves all layers of the bowel
   d. is commonly associated with the formation of fistulas

8. Tony, age 9, has been diagnosed with a peptic ulcer. The nurse includes which one of the following statements in the discharge teaching?

   a. Strict diet therapy must be followed to promote healing of the ulcer.
   b. Administer Carafate on an empty stomach one hour before or two hours after meals.
   c. Administer antacids as prescribed to facilitate healing of the ulcer.
   d. Cure of ulcers is associated with eradication of *E. coli,* the causative organism.

9. The nurse is caring for a preterm, low birth-weight neonate. The following are discovered in the nurse's assessment: abdominal distention, residual gastric contents, feeding intolerance, decreased bowel sounds, and bloody stools. The nurse suspects which condition is most likely occurring?

   a. ulcerative colitis
   b. Crohn's disease
   c. gastroenteritis
   d. necrotizing enterocolitis

10. The nurse is providing preventative health education for a group of school-age children. Good handwashing and proper food handling techniques are emphasized. Which form of hepatitis is best prevented from spread following these practices?

    a. hepatitis A
    b. hepatitis B
    c. hepatitis C
    d. hepatitis D

Multiple Response

1. Sara, age 10 months, had surgical repair for cleft lip and palate. She is being discharged from the acute care facility. When providing family education, the nurse will include which of the following? Select all that apply.

    a. Position Sara on her side.
    b. Offer small amounts of water after feedings to rinse away milk residue.
    c. Remove the elbow restraints several times a day for about 10 minutes.
    d. After feeding, clean the suture line with antibiotic cream.
    e. Position Sara on her back.
    f. Remove restraints at night when Sara sleeps.

2. John is 6 years old. He is seen at the office for repeated problems related to constipation. Dietary teaching provided by the nurse to the family includes which of the following? Select all that apply.

    a. Six-year-olds love macaroni and cheese. I am sure John will love to eat that for you.
    b. Popcorn is a good snack for John to have.
    c. Raisins are a good source of fiber for John.
    d. It would be best for John to eat vegetables that are raw.
    e. Be sure John has plenty of fluids every day.
    f. Bananas are a good food choice for John.

3. Which of the following statements about Celiac disease are true? Select all that apply.

    a. Children will outgrow the disease within 2 years.
    b. Rice is an appropriate dietary component.
    c. People with this condition have stools that float in water.
    d. Rye bread should be consumed instead of white bread.
    e. Corn millet is allowed in the diet of people with this disease.
    f. Absorption problems of Vitamin K exist in individuals with this disease.

4. The nurse should inform the caregivers of a child taking sulfasalazine therapy for the treatment of inflammatory bowel disease to call the health care provider if they experience which of the following? Select all that apply.

   a. yellow-orange skin

   b. yellow-orange urine

   c. skin rash

   d. sore throat

   e. mouth sores

   f. fatigue

Critical Thinking/Case Study

Lowanda is a 3-month-old infant who has recently been diagnosed with gastroesophageal reflux. She was born at 32 weeks' gestation via Cesarean section. Her parents are exhausted. Lowanda is their first child. Mom states, "I feel terrible. Lowanda is just not growing like she should. All she does is cry. She throws up all the time. I am such a bad mother. What did I do to cause this?" Dad is very supportive. He helps care for Lowanda. Dad states, "I have an ulcer. Did I give this to Lowanda, the stomach problem, I mean?" Both parents state they are very confused and scared. They do not know how they will manage to care for Lowanda.

1. What is the incidence and etiology of gastroesophageal reflux?

   _____

   _____

   _____

2. How does gastroesophageal reflux differ from pyloric stenosis?

   _____

   _____

   _____

3. How would you answer the parents' questions about how Lowanda developed this condition and whether they were to blame?

   _____

   _____

   _____

4. What would you include in family teaching? What are the dietary modifications? Positioning techniques? Medications that most likely will be used?

_____

_____

_____

CHAPTER 24

Respiratory Alterations

True or False

1. Small airways, fewer alveoli, and increased chest compliance are leading factors that predispose pediatric populations to respiratory alterations.

   ❑ True   ❑ False

2. Infants are typically mouth breathers.

   ❑ True   ❑ False

3. Frequent swallowing following tonsillectomy is the earliest manifestation of bleeding.

   ❑ True   ❑ False

4. Tonsillectomies are performed on children over 3 years of age, since excessive blood loss is more apt to occur in younger children.

   ❑ True   ❑ False

5. The eustachian tubes of children under the age of 3 years are positioned vertically.

   ❑ True   ❑ False

6. Amoxicillin (Amoxil) is the first-line antibiotic used to treat acute otitis media.

   ❑ True   ❑ False

7. Garlic treats cough and acts as an antibiotic.

   ❑ True   ❑ False

8. Use of TB skin tests as a screening measure for school, camps, or day care for children at low-risk should be discouraged.

   ❑ True   ❑ False

9. Children with allergic rhinitis are also frequently affected by asthma.

   ❑ True   ❑ False

10. The basic underlying pathologic effect of asthma is increased mucus production.

    ❑ True   ❑ False

11. The primary systems affected by cystic fibrosis are the pulmonary and gastrointestinal systems.

    ❑ True   ❑ False

12. Lung transplantation is an end-stage treatment for children with cystic fibrosis.

    ❑ True   ❑ False

13. Bronchopulmonary dysplasia is a chronic lung disease that primarily affects premature infants with respiratory distress syndrome.

    ❑ True   ❑ False

14. Tuberculosis is a viral infection.

    ❑ True   ❑ False

15. The most important finding in the clinical diagnosis of sinusitis is cold symptoms that last longer than three days.

    ❑ True   ❑ False

16. Hypoxemia that is unresponsive to oxygen therapy is a strong indicator of acute respiratory distress syndrome (**ARDS**).

    ❑ True   ❑ False

17. Over-the-counter cough and cold medications for young children are not recommended.

    ❑ True   ❑ False

18. The food most commonly associated with fatal outcomes of foreign body aspirations are hot dogs.

    ❑ True   ❑ False

19. Second-hand smoke increases the number of respiratory infections experienced by children.

    ❑ True   ❑ False

20. Cystic fibrosis is the leading cause of chronic illness in children.

    ❑ True   ❑ False

Fill in the Blank

1. _____ is a term analogous to the common cold.

2. Untreated streptococcal tonsillitis and pharyngitis infections may lead to health problems such as _____, _____, and _____.

3. Treatment for otitis media includes _____, which is a surgical incision in the tympanic membrane for draining fluid.

4. Croup syndrome is manifested by a "barking" cough and inspiratory _____, which is a high-pitched sound produced by an obstruction of the trachea or larynx that can be heard during inspiration and/or expiration.

5. Classic manifestations of acute epiglottitis include: _____, _____, _____, _____, _____, _____, and _____.

6. The classic manifestations of asthma are _____, _____, and _____.

7. Cystic fibrosis is an inherited disorder that affects the _____ glands of the body.

8. In individuals with cystic fibrosis, chronic infection and airway obstruction lead to bronchial epithelium destruction and _____ (a lung condition characterized by irreversible dilation and destruction of the bronchial walls), atelectasis and _____ (a collection of air or gas in the pleural cavity), as well as pulmonary hypertension and _____ (right-sided heart failure).

9. Treatment of the newborn with respiratory distress syndrome includes administration of exogenous _____, which lowers alveolar surface tension, allowing the alveoli to open more easily with inspiration and preventing collapse on expiration.

10. A vaccine that is used for individuals with repeated exposure to tuberculosis is _____.

11. Some of the serious and life-threatening complications from sinusitis that children can develop include: _____, _____, _____, _____, and _____.

12. Premature infants born at less than 36 weeks' gestation may develop _____.

13. _____ is a classic manifestation of bronchiolitis.

14. Some health promotion strategies nurses can implement to reduce the pediatric population's risk for developing respiratory alterations include: _____, _____, _____, _____, and _____.

15. _____ is a pneumonia occurring in a previously healthy child with no underlying condition or disorder or disease outside of the hospital setting.

16. _____ is the only specific therapy for RSV bronchiolitis.

Matching

_____ 1. inhaled nonsteroidal anti-inflammatory

    a. salmeterol

_____ 2. long-acting bronchodilator

    b. prednisolone

_____ 3. antileukotriene

    c. cromolyn

_____ 4. systemic corticosteroid

    d. albuterol sulfate

_____ 5. short-acting beta2-agonists

    e. montelukast sodium

Multiple Choice

1. Which comment by a caregiver of a 7-year-old child with viral nasopharyngitis indicates that further teaching is indicated?

   a. I will have my child gargle with a saline solution.
   b. I will administer over-the-counter antihistamines to my child.
   c. I will administer nonaspirin pain killers and fever reducers to my child as instructed.
   d. I will instill nasal drops for my child.

2. Missy comes to the neighborhood nursing clinic with her 14-month-old daughter Kristen. Missy asks the nurse what can be done to help Kristen, who has a cold. Missy took Kristen to visit the primary care provider the day before and is concerned because Kristen still has a runny nose. Which of the following statements by Missy indicates further teaching is needed?

   a. I insist that my baby receive an antibiotic to treat this infection.
   b. I will make sure that Kristen consumes adequate fluids.
   c. I will position Kristen with her head elevated when she is lying down.
   d. I will use frequent handwashing for myself and following sneezing or nose blowing to deter spread of infection.

3. Mariah is a healthy 5-year-old who is to undergo a tonsillectomy. The nurse needs to include which of the following in the preoperative tests to be ordered for Mariah?

    a. chest X-ray
    b. electrocardiogram
    c. clotting and bleeding times
    d. barium swallow

4. When caring for a child immediately after a tonsillectomy, which action by the new nurse requires immediate intervention by the supervising nurse? The new nurse:

    a. has the child cough and do deep breathing exercises
    b. provides cool humidification
    c. suctions the mouth gently if necessary
    d. positions the child on his or her abdomen or side

5. Nicholas, age 26 months, has acute otitis media. Which statement by his caregiver indicates that more teaching is needed?

    a. I will give Nicholas ibuprofen as prescribed to reduce his pain.
    b. I will offer Nicholas his favorite clear liquids at regular intervals.
    c. I will not use antihistamines and decongestants in his treatment.
    d. I will position Nicholas with his head flat on the affected side to minimize pain.

6. Immediate care of the child with acute epiglottitis includes:

    a. depressing the tongue to view the posterior pharnyx
    b. placing the child in the supine position
    c. thrusting the child's chin back
    d. allowing the child to mouth breathe in the position of comfort

7. Which action by a new nurse caring for a child with acute epiglottitis requires immediate intervention by the supervising nurse? The new nurse:

    a. prepares equipment for a tracheostomy if needed
    b. examines the throat of the child by depressing the tongue
    c. administers antibiotics as prescribed
    d. maintains the child in an upright sitting position

8. Which statement by the caregiver of a child with laryngotracheobronchitis indicates that more teaching is needed?

    a. The other name for laryngotracheobronchitis is croup; it is a common viral syndrome in children between 6 months and 3 years of age.

    b. My child should be given limited amounts of fluids.

    c. It would be best to position my child in the upright position with the head of the bed elevated.

    d. Children with laryngotracheobronchitis commonly receive steroids to help decrease inflammation of the airways.

9. Juan is 9 years old. He has been admitted to the acute care facility with pneumonia. Which action by the student nurse requires intervention by the supervising nurse? The student nurse:

    a. withholds pain medications to prevent respiratory depression

    b. performs chest physiotherapy as indicated

    c. changes Juan's position at least every two hours

    d. administers antibiotics as prescribed

10. Which of the following statements will the nurse include when teaching a group of children and their caregivers about asthma?

    a. Asthma causes airways to become damaged over time as a result of chronic inflammation.

    b. Asthma is characterized by spasms of the trachea.

    c. Pharmacologic management is aimed at reduction of bronchoconstriction.

    d. Asthma is a viral syndrome.

11. Which of the following statements about the pharmacologic management of childhood asthma is true?

    a. Long-acting beta 2-agonists include albuterol.

    b. Inhaled corticosteroids include albuterol sulfate (Proventil).

    c. Antileukotrienes include montelukast.

    d. Inhaled corticosteroids include cromolyn.

12. Which of the following medications is indicated in the treatment of the child with an acute asthma attack?

    a. Zafirlukast (Accolate)
    b. cromolyn
    c. albuterol
    d. salmeterol

Multiple Response

1. Xi, age 3, has just been diagnosed with cystic fibrosis. Her mother asks the nurse what the nurse can tell her about this disease. Which of the following are appropriate responses by the nurse? Select all that apply.

    a. Cystic fibrosis affects the exocrine glands of the body.
    b. The pulmonary system is the primary system affected by the disease.
    c. Cystic fibrosis is usually manifested as an individual experiencing chronic respiratory infections.
    d. The best diet for Xi to be on is high-fat/low-protein.
    e. Most children with cystic fibrosis die between the ages of 10 and 12.
    f. Lung transplantation is contraindicated in children with cystic fibrosis.

2. Which of the following statements about bronchopulmonary dysplasia are true? Select all that apply.

    a. Mechanical ventilation predisposes premature infants to develop bronchopulmonary dysplasia.
    b. Topical administration of steroids to the infant's lungs is the primary treatment for bronchopulmonary dysplasia.
    c. Intravenous surfactant is used to increase lung compliance in the newborn who has bronchopulmonary dysplasia.
    d. Bronchopulmonary dysplasia primarily affects infants who are post-term.
    e. Lung transplantation is the only cure for bronchopulmonary dysplasia.
    f. Bronchopulmonary dysplasia predisposes the individual to lung cancer later on in life.

3. Which of the following statements about tuberculosis are true? Select all that apply.

    a. Tuberculosis is a viral infection.

    b. Tuberculosis is the leading cause of infection-related death in the world.

    c. The transmission of tuberculosis occurs through contact with blood of infected individuals.

    d. A positive Mantoux test is diagnostic of active tuberculosis.

    e. Tuberculosis is a bacterial infection.

    f. A positive sputum culture is diagnostic of active tuberculosis.

4. The nurse identifies common symptoms of cystic fibrosis as which of the following? Select all that apply.

    a. nasal polyps

    b. pancreatitis

    c. hyperproteinemia

    d. respiratory infections by Pseudomonas

    e. black stools

    f. rectal prolapse

Critical Thinking/Case Study

Davona is a nurse who has been asked to present a talk to a group of caregivers of children ages 8 to 12 who have been diagnosed with asthma. Help Davona prepare for this talk by answering the following questions.

1. What would be the best way for Davona to describe the normal anatomy and physiology of the lung? How should Davona describe the effect of asthma on the lung?

    _____

    _____

    _____

2. How could Davona best describe the clinical manifestations of asthma to the caregivers?

    _____

    _____

    _____

3. Most children with asthma have had pulmonary function testing in the diagnostic workup and will continue to have it for follow-up to treatment. Explain pulmonary function testing to the caregivers.

_____

_____

_____

4. Help Davona come up with methods to teach families how to avoid asthma triggers.

_____

_____

_____

5. How would you suggest Davona teach caregivers the technique necessary to assess regular peak expiratory flow monitoring?

_____

_____

_____

6. Multiple studies indicate that most children and families treat asthma only when symptoms are present. How would you suggest Davona teach caregivers about the need to maintain regular consistent administration of controller medications?

_____

_____

_____

7. What would be the most effective method for Davona to use in teaching caregivers pharmacologic treatment of asthma?

_____

_____

_____

8. What should Davona include in education of caregivers on when to take the child with asthma to the primary care provider or emergency department?

_____

_____

_____

CHAPTER 25

Cardiovascular Alterations

True or False

1. When evaluating infants for cardiovascular alterations, feeding behaviors should be assessed because eating is the exercise of the neonate.

   ❏ True   ❏ False

2. Cyanosis is best evaluated under fluorescent lighting.

   ❏ True   ❏ False

3. All murmurs in infants and children are pathologic.

   ❏ True   ❏ False

4. After cardiac catheterization, sandbags should be placed at the catheter site to prevent or treat bleeding.

   ❏ True   ❏ False

5. Systemic venous congestion indicates right ventricular failure.

   ❏ True   ❏ False

6. Peripheral edema in infants is usually localized to the periorbital area.

   ❏ True   ❏ False

7. Diaphoresis is frequently noted during feeding in infants with heart failure.

   ❏ True   ❏ False

8. The approximate size of a child's heart is the size of the child's fist.

   ❏ True   ❏ False

9. In the infant or child with atrial septal defect, blood flows from the right to the left side of the heart across the atrial septal defect.

   ❏ True   ❏ False

10. Surgical repair of an atrial septal defect is usually performed within the first two years of life.

    ❏ True ❏ False

11. The ductus arteriosus is a direct connection between the main pulmonary artery and the aorta.

    ❏ True ❏ False

12. With the advent of penicillin, the incidence of acute rheumatic fever has decreased in the United States.

    ❏ True ❏ False

13. In acute rheumatic fever, the most frequently affected valve is the tricuspid valve.

    ❏ True ❏ False

14. Secondary prophylaxis is essential in the treatment of all individuals with rheumatic carditis and consists of treatment with oral penicillin, 250 mg twice a day, or monthly intramuscular injections of penicillin.

    ❏ True ❏ False

15. African Americans and Asians have higher blood pressure levels than whites.

    ❏ True ❏ False

16. Blood pressure measurements should be performed as part of all routine physical examinations on all children older than 1 year of age.

    ❏ True ❏ False

17. The most common cause of maldistributive shock is sepsis.

    ❏ True ❏ False

18. Nesiritide (Natrecor) is a recombinant brain natriuretic peptide (BNP) given as a continuous infusion to treat severe decompensated congestive heart failure.

    ❏ True ❏ False

19. The cardiovascular system is the first system to function in the developing fetus.

    ❏ True ❏ False

20. Peripheral cyanosis of the extremities is usually caused by vasomotor instability of the young infant.

    ❏ True ❏ False

Fill in the Blank

1. Following birth, _____ and _____ trigger the normal physiologic responses responsible for the transition from fetal to neonatal circulation.

2. _____ is the amount of blood in the ventricle at the end of diastole and just prior to systole. _____ is the resistance that the ventricle must overcome to eject blood.

3. Extreme cyanosis that results in a deep blue or purple color of the entire body is called _____.

4. _____ is the soft tissue deformity that is the result of chronic cyanosis with the subsequent development of the loss of the normal angle between the nail and the nail bed.

5. Medications directed to improve contractility of the heart are referred to as _____.

6. In the premature infant, closure of the patent ductus arteriosus is attempted by the infusion of _____, which inhibits the synthesis of prostaglandin.

7. Truncus arteriosus can be associated with _____, which is a congenital syndrome associated with hypoplasia or aplasia of the thymus and parathyroid glands.

8. In infants with chronic cyanosis, _____ is an adaptive mechanism in which red cell production is increased in an attempt to compensate for decreased oxygen delivery, leading to an increased hematocrit.

9. A(n) _____ involves using a balloon-tipped catheter to dilate a cardiac valve. An incision into a cardiac valve to correct a defect is a(n) _____.

10. Tetralogy of Fallot is made up of four components: _____, _____, _____, and _____.

11. In transposition of the great vessels, the _____ comes off the right ventricle and the _____ comes off the left ventricle.

12. The classic clinical finding in the child with coarctation is _____ and a noticeable difference in blood pressure between the _____.

13. Children who are recipients of artificial valves must be given anticoagulation medications such as _____ to prevent clot formation on the valve.

14. There are some fairly classic skin lesions seen with infective endocarditis. The lesions include _____ and _____.

15. The diagnostic evaluation for a child whose history or physical examination suggests a specific cause of hypertension should be guided by the suspected problem, initially focusing on the _____ system.

16. _____ is the most common arrhythmia seen in infants and children.

17. Generally, shock can be divided into three major classifications: _____, _____, and _____.

18. If a child is in need of blood replacement, until proper typing and cross matching can be performed, _____ should be given.

19. Two ACE inhibitors used in the treatment of children with congestive heart failure include _____ and_____.

Matching

_____ 1. Kawasaki disease

_____ 2. dysmorphic

_____ 3. cardiac tamponade

_____ 4. foramen ovale

_____ 5. desquamation

_____ 6. inotropes

_____ 7. cardiac output

_____ 8. cardioplegia

_____ 9. ductus arteriosus

a. medication directed at improving contractility of the heart

b. blood vessel connecting aorta with the pulmonary artery

c. cessation of cardiac function that follows injection of a cold, high-potassium solution in the heart

d. peeling of skin

e. volume of blood ejected by the heart in one minute

f. larger than normal for age

g. excessive variation in systolic pressure with respiration

h. involuntary purposeless movement of the extremities and trunk

i. abnormal or unusual facial features, edema, chest wall deformities, and skin colors

_____ 10. ectasia

j. accumulation of fluid around the heart that restricts filling of the heart

_____ 11. chorea

k. normal in utero connection in the atrial septum

_____ 12. pulsus paradoxus

l. multisystem vasculitis

Multiple Choice

1. A new nurse is caring for a child who is about to undergo a cardiac catheterization. Which action by the new nurse requires the supervising nurse to intervene? The new nurse:

   a. determines history of latex allergy
   b. obtains base-line pedal pulses and pulse oximetry
   c. ensures that the child eats a meal just prior to the procedure
   d. reviews laboratory results including platelet count

2. Josh, age 5, has just returned to the floor after having a cardiac catheterization. The insertion site was his right groin. Which one of the following interventions will the nurse perform?

   a. Position Josh in high Fowler's.
   b. Encourage Josh to walk in the halls one hour after the procedure.
   c. Place a sandbag at the area of Josh's right groin.
   d. Assist with removal of the pressure dressing in 24 hours.

3. Suzette is a 2-month-old infant with congestive heart failure. The nurse teaches Suzette's mother why nutritional support is critically important in the infant with congestive heart failure. Which statement by Suzette's mother indicates that more teaching is needed?

   a. I will limit feedings and calories to prevent Suzette from gaining unwanted weight.
   b. I will add less water to the concentrate or powder to increase the number of calories.
   c. Some babies with congestive heart failure have a tube inserted from the nose to the stomach or intestine to administer feedings.
   d. I will add calories to Suzette's feedings by gradually increasing them over a number of days.

4. Suzette, a 2-month-old infant with congestive heart failure, is being discharged from the acute care center. Which one of the following is included by the nurse in discharge teaching to Suzette's family?

   a. Expect Suzette to have some difficulty breathing as she adjusts to the new home environment.

   b. All individuals caring for Suzette need to be taught cardiopulmonary resuscitation.

   c. To conserve Suzette's energy, allow infrequent, longer periods of time for feedings.

   d. All medications will be administered by the home health nurse. Don't worry about them. Just keep them filled.

5. Emily is a 9-month-old with tetralogy of Fallot. As the nurse is assessing her, Emily goes into a hypercyanotic spell. The nurse should:

   a. administer morphine

   b. institute volume resuscitation to decrease blood viscosity

   c. hold Emily in an upright position to facilitate expansion of the lungs

   d. place Emily in the knee-chest position

6. Joaquim, age 8, is being discharged from the acute care facility after repair of a congenital heart defect. Which statement by Joaquim's caregiver indicates that more teaching is needed?

   a. Joaquim may return to school within approximately two weeks.

   b. For the first week after discharge, I will have Joaquim soak in a bathtub with the chest incision submerged under water.

   c. Joaquim may follow a regular diet.

   d. I will call my primary care provider if Joaquim develops puffiness of the eyes, swelling of the feet, shortness of breath, or excessive irritability.

7. George, age 9, has been diagnosed with acute rheumatic fever. The nurse expects George to receive which one of the following medications as standard treatment for this condition?

   a. intravenous penicillin

   b. aspirin

   c. acetaminophen

   d. ibuprofen

8. Elaine is the mother of 12-year-old Brandon who has been diagnosed with hypertension. Elaine asks the nurse, "How can this be possible? Brandon is only a child. He can't possibly have high blood pressure. The doctor is wrong. What can you tell me about high blood pressure in kids?" The best response for the nurse to make is:

   a. Children with high blood pressure are at a very high risk for death. The doctor is right. Brandon needs treatment.

   b. Maybe Brandon has a problem with his liver. Often if the liver problem is corrected, the high blood pressure is also corrected.

   c. The most effective method for a 12-year-old to lose weight is to lower excessive caloric intake and to increase physical exercise. Weight reduction usually results in lower blood pressure readings.

   d. For children with hypertension, medication administration is the most effective method to lower their blood pressure.

9. Which of the following statements about cardiac transplantation in the pediatric population is true?

   a. The major roadblock to transplantation at this time is the lack of technologic support.

   b. The child who receives a heart transplant will be on antirejection medications for the first year after the transplant, after which time the medication is discontinued.

   c. Children waiting for a cardiac transplant are listed by their body mass index.

   d. Long-term complications of cardiac transplant include the development of coronary artery disease requiring retransplantation.

10. Priority nursing care for the child experiencing anaphylaxis is:

    a. Notify the parents.
    b. Secure an airway.
    c. Find the cause of the reaction.
    d. Obtain a blood pressure.

Multiple Response

1. The nurse recognizes which of the following as components of the Jones criteria for diagnosis of acute rheumatic fever? Select all that apply.

   a. pneumococcal infection
   b. fever
   c. arthralgia
   d. polyarthritis
   e. positive Jones antibodies
   f. leukopenia

2. The nurse has been asked to speak with a group of parents whose children have Kawasaki disease. When explaining the pathophysiology, the nurse includes which of the following statements? Select all that apply.

   a. In the early stage of the illness, the heart is inflamed.
   b. The specific cause of the disease is not known.
   c. Kawasaki disease results in localized inflammation of blood vessels of the child's brain.
   d. The most characteristic finding of this disease is changes of the hands and feet.
   e. Vasculitis occurs most frequently in the gastrointetinal system.
   f. Aneurysms occur most frequently in the Circle of Willis.

3. Edwin is 7 years old. He is being discharged from the acute care facility with a permanent pacemaker. In providing discharge teaching for Edwin and his parents, the nurse includes which of the following statements? Select all that apply.

   a. Edwin may never have an MRI scan.
   b. Keep Edwin away from microwave ovens.
   c. If Edwin uses a cell phone, have him use it on the opposite side of the generator.
   d. Have Edwin avoid contact sports.
   e. Edwin will not be able to travel in an airplane because he cannot go through security.
   f. Edwin should avoid spending a lot of time in power plants.

4. An 8-year-old child is admitted to the emergency department with supraventricular tachycardia. The nurse expects which of the following interventions to be used to treat the child? Select all that apply.

   a. Ask the child to breathe rapidly.

   b. Administer intravenous adenosine.

   c. Ask the child to bear down as if having a bowel movement.

   d. Monitor immediate cardioversion.

   e. Ask the child to do a head stand.

   f. Administer intravenous lidocaine.

Critical Thinking/Case Study

Rosaria is 1 month old. She has been diagnosed with cardiomyopathy and congestive heart failure. Rosaria's caregivers ask the nurse several questions. How could the nurse best respond to the following questions?

1. I don't understand how a baby's heart can just not work well. What is the problem with Rosaria's heart? She is just a baby; how can her heart be damaged? She didn't have a heart attack, did she?

   _____

   _____

   _____

2. I feel so bad when Rosaria wants to eat. She seems to get so upset. Why does my baby have such a hard time with sucking? What can I do to help Rosaria get the milk I know she wants and needs?

   _____

   _____

   _____

3. The doctor said my little Rosaria has to take a water pill, furosemide (Lasix), and another pill, digoxin (Lanoxin). My grandmother takes these same pills for her heart. Why does my baby have to take such pills?

_____

_____

_____

CHAPTER 26

Hematological Alterations

True or False

1. Anemia is the most common blood disorder in children.

   ❑ True   ❑ False

2. If a child experiences sequestration crisis frequently, a splenectomy may be performed.

   ❑ True   ❑ False

3. Breast milk should be encouraged as the exclusive source of nutrition in infants because the bioavailability of iron in human milk is greater than that of iron-fortified formulas.

   ❑ True   ❑ False

4. When a child is receiving iron supplements, one way to tell if the child is getting enough iron is that his or her stools will be a tarry black color.

   ❑ True   ❑ False

5. The sickle cell trait is associated with decreased life expectancy.

   ❑ True   ❑ False

6. The principal symptom experienced by children with sickle cell anemia is pain.

   ❑ True   ❑ False

7. In the United States, sickle cell anemia is more prevalent in the African-American population.

   ❑ True   ❑ False

8. The beta-Thalassemias are common among children of Mediterranean descent.

   ❑ True   ❑ False

9. A splenectomy is often performed on children with thalassemia major to eliminate the site of hemolysis, which can decrease the child's need for frequent transfusions.

   ❑ True   ❑ False

10. Aplastic anemia is a condition in which injury to or abnormal expression of stem cells in bone marrow results in inadequate numbers of erythrocytes while numbers of leukocytes and platelets remain normal.

    ❑ True   ❑ False

11. The only potential cure for Fanconi's anemia is bone marrow transplant.

    ❑ True   ❑ False

12. Disseminated intravascular coagulation (DIC) is a coagulation disorder in which the stimulus for coagulation is not present.

    ❑ True   ❑ False

13. Von Willebrand's disease is the most common congenital disorder of homeostasis.

    ❑ True   ❑ False

Fill in the Blank

1. Production of red blood cells is called _____, while destruction of red blood cells is referred to as _____.

2. In children of all ages, dietary iron is absorbed in the small intestine and either passed into the bloodstream or stored in the intestinal epithelial cells as _____.

3. The recommended form of oral iron supplementation is _____ iron because it is the most efficiently absorbed.

4. The term _____ refers to the aggregation of sickled cells within a vessel, causing obstruction.

5. The term _____ refers to the excessive pooling of blood in the liver and spleen.

6. _____ is a group of inherited autosomal recessive disorders, characterized by an impaired rate of hemoglobin chain synthesis.

7. Repeated blood transfusions can result in a buildup of excess iron in the body, causing iron overload or _____.

8. A _____ is a drug that is used to either prevent or reverse the toxic effects of a heavy metal or to accelerate the elimination of the metal from the body.

9. _____ are pockets of blood under the skin caused by excessive bleeding following trauma.

10. _____ refers to a condition in which all three types of blood cells are either decreased or absent.

11. The _____ are a group of bleeding disorders in which one factor in the first phase of coagulation is deficient.

12. Children with hemophilia often experience bleeding into the joints, which is referred to as _____.

Matching

_____ 1. hemolysis

_____ 2. hemostasis

_____ 3. sequestration crisis

_____ 4. Desferal

_____ 5. sickle cell anemia

_____ 6. erythropoietin

_____ 7. hemosiderosis

_____ 8. aplastic crisis

a. control of bleeding

b. stimulation of red blood cell production

c. iron overdose

d. excessive pooling of blood in the liver and spleen

e. buildup of excessive iron in the blood

f. decreased erythropoiesis

g. destruction of red blood cells

h. hemoglobin S

Multiple Choice

1. The presence of which vitamin is most effective in enhancing absorption of iron?

    a. vitamin A

    b. vitamin B

    c. vitamin C

    d. vitamin D

2. Which one of the following children with sickle cell anemia is at greatest risk for exacerbation of the disease?

    a. Anita, who lives in Pittsburgh and is visiting Denver, Colorado, to go snow skiing

    b. Jacques, who is spending a warm summer day swimming with his friends

    c. Ed, who is learning how to roller blade

    d. Janessa, who is in a gymnastics class

3. Takisha, age 8, has been admitted to the hospital in sickle cell crisis. She complains of pain all over her body. Which intervention by the new nurse requires the supervising nurse to intervene? The new nurse:

   a. allows Takisha to determine the level of activity she can tolerate
   b. provides Takisha passive range of motion exercises
   c. administers fluids to maintain hydration status
   d. applies ice packs to specific painful areas of the body

4. In a child with beta-thalassemia major, the nurse would expect to find which of the following clinical manifestations?

   a. long thin nose
   b. malocclusion
   c. narrow set eyes
   d. concave forehead

5. The first line of treatment for type I, or mild type II, von Willebrand's disease is:

   a. desmopressin
   b. heparin
   c. warfarin sodium (Coumadin)
   d. protamine

6. Which of the following over-the-counter medications should not be taken by a child who has immune thrombocytopenic purpura?

   a. ibuprofen (Motrin)
   b. aspirin
   c. acetaminophen (Tylenol)
   d. ibuprofen (Advil)

7. The child with disseminated intravascular coagulation is at greatest risk for the development of which complication?

   a. infection
   b. airway obstruction
   c. hemorrhage
   d. impaired skin integrity

8. A caregiver of a child with a bleeding disorder has been taught the actions to take for treatment of a nosebleed. Which statement by the caregiver indicates that more teaching is needed? If the child experiences a nosebleed I will:

   a. lie the child down
   b. pinch the child's nose
   c. hold the nose for at least 10 minutes
   d. apply ice to the bridge of the nose

9. Which of the following is considered appropriate treatment for hemophilia B?

   a. factor VIII concentrates
   b. Desmopressin
   c. aspirin
   d. factor IX concentrates

10. Which of the following is a side effect associated with cyclosporine therapy for the treatment of aplastic anemia?

    a. decreased blood pressure
    b. loss of body hair
    c. gingival hyperplasia
    d. decreased potassium

Multiple Response

1. Which of the following are compensatory mechanisms for anemia? Select all that apply.

   a. increased erythropoiesis
   b. decreased heart rate
   c. retention of sodium
   d. increased respiratory rate
   e. retention of water
   f. leukocytosis

2. Marty, age 14, has iron deficiency anemia. When talking with him about which types of foods to choose that are high in iron content, the nurse suggests which of the following? Select all that apply.

    a. peas

    b. potatoes

    c. bananas

    d. peaches

    e. raisins

    f. shrimp

3. Initial signs and symptoms of iron overdose include which of the following? Select all that apply.

    a. skin rash

    b. vomiting

    c. abdominal pain

    d. bloody diarrhea

    e. lethargy

    f. dyspnea

4. Which of the following are stimuli for sickle cell crisis? Select all that apply.

    a. exposure to heat

    b. infection

    c. fever

    d. acidosis

    e. diet high in carbohydrates

    f. immunizations

Critical Thinking/Case Study

Jared, a student nurse, has been asked by his clinical instructor to design a poster about sickle cell anemia to be displayed at a community wellness fair that will be sponsored by the school of nursing. What would be the most effective method for Jared to use in designing the poster? He will be present at the poster display as people walk by. Help Jared with his project by answering the following questions.

1. What information should be included on the poster about the incidence and etiology of sickle cell anemia?

   _____

   _____

   _____

2. Jared plans to develop a diagram illustrating the pathophysiology of sickle cell anemia. What would be the most effective way to represent the clinical manifestations of sickle cell anemia—pictures, written descriptions, or something else?

   _____

   _____

   _____

3. A participant at the health fair asks Jared what the treatment options are for sickle cell anemia. How should Jared answer this question?

   _____

   _____

   _____

CHAPTER 27

Immunologic Alterations

True or False

1. The immune system of neonates and young children is immature.

   ❑ True   ❑ False

2. Presently there is no cure for systemic lupus erythematosus.

   ❑ True   ❑ False

3. Diagnosis of juvenile idiopathic arthritis is made by thorough history and physical assessment findings.

   ❑ True   ❑ False

4. Application of cold packs to the joints of children with juvenile idiopathic arthritis is damaging.

   ❑ True   ❑ False

5. Juvenile idiopathic arthritis is the most common pediatric rheumatologic disease.

   ❑ True   ❑ False

6. Approximately 70% of individuals with juvenile rheumatoid arthritis experience permanent remissions and function optimally.

   ❑ True   ❑ False

7. Onset of systemic lupus erythematosus in childhood usually occurs before the age of 2.

   ❑ True   ❑ False

8. Pregnancy is not possible in individuals with systemic lupus erythematosus.

   ❑ True   ❑ False

9. Chronic otitis media, thrush, and pneumocystis carinii pneumonia are infections common in HIV-infected infants even before they are diagnosed with HIV.

   ❑ True   ❑ False

10. Infants cannot become infected with HIV through breast milk.

    ❑ True   ❑ False

11. In general, the younger a child is at the time of acquisition of HIV, the more severe the symptoms, the more quickly the disease progresses, and the poorer the prognosis.

    ❑ True   ❑ False

12. The standard ELISA HIV antibody test can be used on infants.

    ❑ True   ❑ False

13. The World Health Organization now considers HIV/AIDS as a chronic illness that can be managed.

    ❑ True   ❑ False

14. HIV affects all systems of the body.

    ❑ True   ❑ False

Fill in the Blank

1. _____ is the identification of self as non-self.

2. _____ is specific immunity, triggered when a person has had prior contact with a foreign agent.

3. _____ refers to the passing or administration of preformed antibodies to someone.

4. A term used to describe a condition in which the child's immune system has become so compromised that one of the many diagnoses associated with advanced HIV disease may occur is _____.

5. There has been a significant decrease in morbidity and mortality associated with HIV/AIDS in recent years because of the availability of _____ therapy.

6. A positive result on the ELISA is confirmed by the _____, which identifies particular proteins and glycoproteins found in antibodies specific to HIV.

7. The medication _____ is used as prophylaxis against pneumocystis carinii pneumonia.

8. _____ rashes are the most common form of cutaneous drug reactions.

Matching

_____ 1. complement

_____ 2. immediate hypersensitivity

_____ 3. B lymphocytes

_____ 4. autoimmunity

_____ 5. T lymphocytes

_____ 6. interferons

_____ 7. interleukins

a. inhibits replication of many viruses and has antitumor effects

b. release of chemical mediator such as histamine, or damage to tissue by lysosomal enzymes; short duration between exposure and reaction

c. identification of self is sometimes made as foreign

d. immune system's main defense against viruses

e. 25 serum proteins activated by the onset of the immune response or chemical markers on a pathogen surface

f. produced in the bone marrow and differentiated by five major classes of immunoglobulins: IgG, IgM, IgA, IgE, and IgD

g. chemical mediators that communicate throughout the immune process

Multiple Choice

1. The first-line treatment for juvenile idiopathic arthritis is:

   a. steroids
   b. nonsteroidal anti-inflammatory drugs
   c. aspirin
   d. etanercept (Enbrel)

2. The nurse has provided teaching for the caregivers of a child who is taking steroid therapy. Which statement by the caregiver indicates that more teaching is needed?

   a. My child will gain weight.
   b. My child will exhibit a round face.
   c. My child's blood pressure will decrease.
   d. My child will develop a buffalo hump.

3. Which of the following medications used to control inflammation has a common side effect of retinopathy?

   a. nonsteroidal anti-inflammatory agents

   b. methotrexate

   c. cytotoxics

   d. hydroxychloroquine

4. A mother who is HIV positive asks the nurse when she will know if her baby was infected by the HIV virus. The best response by the nurse is to tell the mother that the waiting period to determine the infection status of the infant is about:

   a. two months

   b. four months

   c. six months

   d. eight months

5. For anaphylaxis, the nurse anticipates administration of which medication as the first drug of choice for treatment of this medical emergency?

   a. diphenhydramine HCL (Benadryl)

   b. epinephrine

   c. lidocaine

   d. morphine

6. For a child experiencing an acute drug reaction, it is most important for the nurse to:

   a. provide good oral hygiene and skin care

   b. teach the child about the treatments ordered and experienced

   c. teach the child and caregivers about the drugs that should be avoided

   d. ensure presence of an effective airway

7. The nurse correctly documents a wheal-like skin lesion as:

   a. urticaria

   b. angioedema

   c. erythema multiforme

   d. maculopapular rash

Multiple Response

1. Which of the following lab results are expected in a child with juvenile idiopathic arthritis? Select all that apply.

   a. increased platelet count
   b. decreased hemoglobin
   c. decreased erythrocyte sedimentation rate
   d. increased white blood cell count
   e. increased potassium
   f. increased BUN

2. Which of the following statements about immunizations of children with HIV are true? Select all that apply.

   a. Children with HIV should receive an annual influenza vaccine.
   b. Following the usual schedule of immunizations is recommended with few exceptions.
   c. Children with HIV should receive the activated form of the polio vaccine.
   d. Children with very low CD4 counts should not receive the varicella vaccine.
   e. Children with very low CD4 counts should receive the measles vaccine.
   f. After any immunization a child with HIV must remain in isolation for at least seven days.

3. Children with HIV experience altered nutrition related to which of the following? Select all that apply.

   a. decreased metabolic rate
   b. stress
   c. anorexia
   d. decreased ability to absorb nutrients
   e. low blood sugars associated with the disease
   f. constant metallic taste resulting from effects of the disease process

Critical Thinking/Case Study

A group of student nurses has been assigned to provide a talk about HIV and AIDS for PTA members at a local junior high school.

1. How should the student nurses define HIV versus AIDS?

   _____

   _____

   _____

2. What common myths and misconceptions about HIV and AIDS should the students address?

_____

_____

_____

3. One of the PTA members tells the student nurses that her son cannot possibly get HIV or AIDS because he is not gay. How should the nurses respond?

_____

_____

_____

4. Another PTA member states that he feels any child with HIV or AIDS should be banned from school. He is asking for the student nurses' support of his position. What would be their best response?

_____

_____

_____

5. How should the nursing students present treatment modalities of HIV and AIDS to the group?

_____

_____

_____

6. One woman states that her daughter who is HIV positive is pregnant. She asks the student nurses if her grandchild will be infected. How should they reply?

_____

_____

_____

CHAPTER 28

Endocrine Alterations

True or False

1. In most children, endocrine disorders are caused by insufficient production of hormones.

   ❏ True   ❏ False

2. At birth, the endocrine system is less mature than any other body system.

   ❏ True   ❏ False

3. Cortisol is the most important mineralocorticoid causing sodium retention and potassium excretion.

   ❏ True   ❏ False

4. Children with precocious puberty have an advanced bone age.

   ❏ True   ❏ False

5. Precocious puberty is treated with a GnRH analog.

   ❏ True   ❏ False

6. A child with hyperkalemia is most at risk for seizure.

   ❏ True   ❏ False

7. The treatment of choice for diabetes insipidus is desmopressin acetate (DDAVP).

   ❏ True   ❏ False

8. Babies with congenital hypothyroidism are generally hyperthermic.

   ❏ True   ❏ False

9. When given in physiologic doses, levothyroxine sodium (Synthroid) has severe side effects.

   ❏ True   ❏ False

10. To maximize absorption, L-thyroxine should be taken with iron.

    ❏ True   ❏ False

11. Adrenarche refers to excessive body hair in a masculine distribution pattern.

    ❑ True   ❑ False

12. No insulin is compatible when mixed in the same syringe with insulin glargine injection (Lantus).

    ❑ True   ❑ False

13. Insulin regimens that utilize a long-acting insulin like insulin glargine injection (Lantus) or use an insulin pump are more physiologic, with a better approximation of normal beta-cell insulin secretion when compared with a 2–3 injection-per-day routine.

    ❑ True   ❑ False

14. Type 1 diabetes is a new epidemic among children and adolescents that results from insulin resistance.

    ❑ True   ❑ False

Fill in the Blank

1. A _____ is a chemical substance produced by an endocrine gland that is secreted into the bloodstream and affects other tissues or organs.

2. The anterior pituitary secretes _____ that cause target tissues to produce hormones.

3. The production of the thyroid hormones is dependent on sufficient dietary intake of _____ and _____ in food and water.

4. The three target organs of parathyroid hormone consist of _____, _____, and _____.

5. Some clinical manifestations of children with growth hormone deficiency include _____ voice, _____ in the trunk area, face that is _____, and a _____ weight for _____ ratio.

6. A _____ is an intramuscular injection of a medication that is absorbed over an extended period of time.

7. When administered at physiologic replacement doses, side effects of growth hormone can include _____, _____, _____, and _____.

8. Precocious puberty is defined as breast development before the age of _____ years in Caucasian girls and before _____ years in African-American girls. In boys less

than _____ years of age, the development of secondary sex characteristics is considered precocity.

9. Sexual maturation staging is also known as _____.

10. _____ is the excretion of an abnormally large amount of urine, and _____ is excessive thirst.

11. The early detection and treatment of hypothyroidism can prevent _____, or severe mental retardation.

12. The most common cause of hyperthyroidism in pediatrics is _____.

13. _____ is bulging of the eyeballs, and proptosis is downward displacement of the eyeball.

14. The development of sexual characteristics of the male in a female is called _____.

15. When a newborn has ambiguous genitalia, the condition is called _____.

16. For children with 21-OH deficiency, gender misidentification is problematic only for the _____.

Matching

_____ 1. secreted by the anterior pituitary

_____ 2. vasopressin

_____ 3. NIDDM

_____ 4. Addison's disease

_____ 5. diabetes insipidus

_____ 6. polyphagia

_____ 7. Cushing's syndrome

_____ 8. hyperthyroidism

_____ 9. Chvostek's sign

_____ 10. pseudohermaphroditism

_____ 11. polydipsia

_____ 12. Trousseau's sign

_____ 13. secreted by the adrenal medulla

_____ 14. IDDM

a. ambiguous genitalia

b. Graves' disease

c. Type I diabetes

d. hypercortisolism

e. norepinephrine

f. excessive thirst

g. Type II diabetes

h. antidiuretic hormone

i. carpopedal spasm

j. growth hormone

k. disorder of water regulation

l. excessive hunger

m. facial muscle spasm

n. hypoadrenal function

Multiple Choice

1. A student nurse is obtaining a height for an 18-month old infant. Which action by the student nurse requires the supervising nurse to intervene? The student nurse:

   a. records the child's height to the nearest full inch
   b. uses the supine position to measure the child's height
   c. places the soles of the child's feet in a 90-degree angle to the footboard
   d. measures the child when the child is barefoot

2. Which statement by a parent of a child receiving growth hormone replacement therapy indicates that more teaching is needed? I will call the primary care provider immediately if my child experiences:

   a. rapid weight gain
   b. headaches
   c. nausea
   d. painful hip joints

3. Which of the following interventions should the nurse follow when administering a medication intranasally?

   a. Have the child lie on the same side where the medication was administered for several minutes after the medication is given.
   b. Have the child lie on the opposite side of where the medication was administered for several minutes after the medication is given.
   c. Have the child blow his or her nose after administering the medication.
   d. Ask the child if he or she swallowed the medication, as this indicates that the medication will be absorbed.

4. Maria, age 6, has been diagnosed with hyperthyroidism. The nurse would expect Maria to exhibit which clinical manifestation?

   a. bradycardia
   b. proptosis
   c. cool skin
   d. drowsiness

5. Which statement by the caregiver of a child with hyperthyroidism indicates that more teaching is needed? Because my child has hyperthyroidism, she will need to be treated with:

    a. thyroid transplant

    b. subtotal thyroidectomy

    c. radioactive iodine therapy

    d. antithyroid medication

6. The nurse is working with a newborn with a diagnosis of pseudohermaphrodism. The nurse should avoid doing which of the following interventions?

    a. Address the newborn with ambiguous genitalia as "it".

    b. Encourage the parents to determine the gender of the baby as soon as possible.

    c. Administer cortisone as prescribed.

    d. Describe the sex organs of the newborn as the penis until corrective surgery can take place.

7. The nurse is teaching children with diabetes mellitus and their families about insulin administration. The nurse informs these individuals that the name of intermediate acting insulin is:

    a. insulin lispro (Humalog)

    b. NPH

    c. insulin (Ultralente)

    d. Regular

8. William is 5 years old. He is taking insulin therapy to manage his diabetes mellitus. According to the developmental target ages for technical skill training in diabetes management, the nurse should expect William to be able to be responsible for which one of the following skills?

    a. insulin dosage adjustment

    b. insulin injections

    c. blood testing

    d. nutrition decision making

9. Matthew is 13 years old. He has just been diagnosed with diabetes mellitus. Matthew is learning how to perform blood glucose testing. Which statement by Matthew indicates that more teaching is needed?

   a. I will use the tip of my finger to obtain the blood specimen.
   b. I will use areas of my fingers with calluses to obtain the blood specimen when possible.
   c. I will warm my fingers before obtaining the blood specimen.
   d. I will wash my hands with soap and water before obtaining the blood specimen.

10. When discussing hypoglycemia with a 10-year-old child with diabetes mellitus and the child's caregivers, which of the following statements by the nurse is true?

    a. Hypoglycemia occurs when the blood sugar is at 90 mg/dL.
    b. Hypoglycemia is caused by less insulin being available than is necessary.
    c. The most common symptoms include drowsiness, lightheadedness, irritability, tremors, sweating, and confusion.
    d. Severe hypoglycemia is a common complication of diabetes that most children experience on a regular basis.

11. A 10-year-old child has been taught about signs and symptoms of hyperglycemia. Which response by the child indicates that more teaching is needed? If I experience hyperglycemia, I will most likely have:

    a. an inability to urinate
    b. a heart beat that is really slow
    c. no desire to drink
    d. fruity odor to my breath

12. A student nurse is preparing to teach a class to senior-level nursing students regarding type 2 diabetes in children. Which statement included in the student's notes requires the faculty to intervene? The student's notes state:

    a. Diabetes is a complex metabolic disorder.
    b. Diabetes is a genetic disease.
    c. Typically, the child with type 2 diabetes is underweight at the time of diagnosis.
    d. The target cells in the body resist insulin stimulated glucose uptake, resulting in hyperinsulinism or insulin resistance.

13. Which one of the following statements should the nurse include in teaching a 12-year-old and his family about metformin HCL (Glucaphage)?

    a. Glucophage is an injectable form of antidiabetic medication.
    b. Glucophage increases insulin production.
    c. Glucophage is indicated for the treatment of adults only.
    d. Glucophage does not cause hypoglycemia.

14. Jeremy is an 8-year-old boy admitted to the pediatric intensive care unit with a diagnosis of diabetic ketoacidosis. Which intervention by the new nurse requires the supervising nurse to intervene? The new nurse:

    a. withholds all insulin, as too much insulin is the cause of the problem
    b. rehydrates Jeremy with fluids to prevent or treat hypovolemic shock
    c. infuses bicarbonate as prescribed
    d. assesses Jeremy for clinical manifestations of cerebral edema

15. Missy is a 1-month-old infant girl who has just been diagnosed with hypoparathyroidism. Missy's mother asks the nurse, "The doctor told me Missy has something wrong with her parathyroid gland. I don't know what this means. Can you tell me about what is going on with my baby and what is being done to help her?" Which statement by the student nurse requires the supervising nurse to intervene?

    a. The main function of the hormone your daughter is missing is to regulate serum potassium.
    b. Missy will be evaluated for bone deformities and limited growth as she develops.
    c. Calcium supplementation will be a major component of Missy's treatment.
    d. Missy will be assessed for seizures or tetany as an acute complication of her hormone deficiency.

Multiple Response

1. Megan is a 2-day-old infant with congenital hypothyroidism. The nurse would expect Megan to exhibit which of the following clinical manifestations of congenital hypothyroidism? Select all that apply.

   a. umbilical hernia
   b. constipation
   c. prolonged jaundice
   d. hyperthermia
   e. sunken eyelids
   f. hypertonia

2. When providing teaching to the caregivers of a child with congenital hypothyroidism, the nurse includes which of the following? Select all that apply.

   a. You can expect your child to receive thyroid replacement therapy for the rest of his (or her) life.
   b. Mix the thyroid replacement medication with soy-based formula products to maximize absorption.
   c. Do not put the crushed pill of thyroid replacement medication in a full bottle of formula.
   d. Keep all appointments for blood tests to evaluate function of the thyroid.
   e. Administer thyroid replacement medications with iron to enhance absorption.
   f. Do not administer the medications on weekends because the child needs a drug holiday to prevent complications.

3. Which of the following are clinical manifestation of acquired hypothyroidism? Select all that apply.

   a. cold intolerance
   b. constipation
   c. weight loss
   d. delayed deep tendon reflexes
   e. edema of the face
   f. delayed puberty

4. The child with Type 1 diabetes most commonly presents with which of the following clinical manifestations? Select all that apply.

   a. polyuria
   b. polydipsia
   c. polyphagia
   d. polyarthralgia
   e. weight loss
   f. dehydration

5. When assessing a child with Cushing's syndrome, the nurse would expect which of the following clinical manifestations? Select all that apply.

   a. buffalo hump
   b. bruising
   c. weight loss
   d. hirsutism
   e. butterfly rash on the face
   f. clubbing of fingers

Critical Thinking/Case Study

Mercedes is a student nurse who has been assigned a project by her clinical instructor. Mercedes has been asked to develop educational classes for a group of children newly diagnosed with diabetes mellitus. The children are 8 to 12 years of age. Assist Mercedes in completing this assignment.

1. How should Mercedes explain to these children the cause of diabetes and how diabetes affects their bodies?

   _____

   _____

   _____

2. Would it be a good idea for Mercedes to separate those children who have Type 1 diabetes from those with Type 2 diabetes for the classes?

_____

_____

_____

3. The classes are for children with diabetes mellitus. How can Mercedes let the caregivers know what information has been taught to the children? Should the caregivers be part of these classes?

_____

_____

_____

4. What would be the most effective way for Mercedes to teach the children about the various types of insulin?

_____

_____

_____

5. The children have already learned how to monitor their blood glucose. What highlights on this technique should Mercedes review with the group?

_____

_____

_____

6. Help Mercedes plan a review of proper insulin administration techniques for these children.

_____

_____

_____

7. Assist Mercedes in developing a creative way to teach the children about the symptoms and actions to take for hypoglycemia and hyperglycemia.

_____

_____

_____

8. What would be an effective method for Mercedes to use in assessing psychosocial implications of diabetes mellitus on the children's lifestyle?

_____

_____

_____

Cellular Alterations

True or False

1. A tumor is a malignant mass.

   ❑ True   ❑ False

2. Lymphoma is an example of a localized cancer.

   ❑ True   ❑ False

3. Chemotherapy is the most frequently used treatment modality in pediatric oncology.

   ❑ True   ❑ False

4. A platelet count of less than 45,000/cu. mm poses a high risk of spontaneous bleeding.

   ❑ True   ❑ False

5. If a child with neutropenia and fever is treated with IV antibiotics and the fever does not subside, and if the causative organism has not been isolated, it may be necessary to start an antifungal agent.

   ❑ True   ❑ False

6. Children who are neutropenic will not mount an immune response to infection.

   ❑ True   ❑ False

7. Giving chemotherapy in the morning may alleviate nausea and vomiting in children.

   ❑ True   ❑ False

8. Children undergoing chemotherapy have fragile intestinal mucosa and should not receive anything per rectum.

   ❑ True   ❑ False

9. Adolescent females on chemotherapy should be encouraged to use tampons as a method to decrease risk of infection.

   ❑ True   ❑ False

10. Leukemia is a term used to describe malignant disease of the thrombocytes.

    ❑ True   ❑ False

11. The treatment goal for leukemia in the induction phase is to reduce the tumor burden to an undetectable level, a state known as remission.

    ❑ True   ❑ False

12. Leukemia cells cannot cross the blood brain barrier.

    ❑ True   ❑ False

13. Hodgkins' disease usually originates in a cervical lymph node.

    ❑ True   ❑ False

14. Hematopoietic stem cell transplantation (HSCT) was previously known as bone marrow transplantation.

    ❑ True   ❑ False

15. Hair loss from chemotherapy is permanent.

    ❑ True   ❑ False

16. The effects of cancer treatment are more severe on male fertility than female fertility.

    ❑ True   ❑ False

Fill in the Blank

1. The most common cancer diagnosed in children is _____.

2. _____ care is given to relieve pain and improve quality of life when cancer treatment is no longer effective.

3. Chemotherapy drugs are classified into six major categories according to their chemical structure: _____, _____, _____, _____, _____, and _____.

4. _____ is the cornerstone of infection prevention and control when working with the child who is neutropenic.

5. Children receiving cyclophosphamide (Cytoxan) and ifosfamide (Ifex) are at risk for _____ (abnormal bleeding of the bladder), which may occur during the administration of the agent or months afterward.

6. When working with clients who have received chemotherapy, nurses need to take precautions for _____ after single-agent chemotherapy and _____ after multiagent chemotherapy.

7. Examples of biologic response modifiers include: _____, _____, _____, and _____.

8. _____ (a biological response modifier) are produced in the laboratory to target cancer cells. They are used to deliver immunotoxins, detect cancer in the early stages, and deliver radioactive isotopes.

9. _____ is a natural human protein produced by the body in small amounts and is capable of inhibiting viral replication, modulating immune responses, and altering cellular proliferation.

10. Once chemotherapy begins, the release of purines from the destroyed leukemic lymphoblasts causes an elevation of uric acid that can lead to acute renal failure. This is called _____.

11. Some chemotherapy drugs are _____ or skin irritating and cause discomfort with sensations of burning, redness, and inflammation if they _____ or leak out of the vein during administration.

12. _____ is the implantation of radioactive "seeds" or "pellets" directly into a body cavity, skin surface, or tissue.

13. Osteosarcoma treatment includes _____ of the affected bone.

Matching

_____ 1. xerostomia

_____ 2. pancytopenia

_____ 3. purpura

_____ 4. alopecia

_____ 5. ataxia

_____ 6. petechiae

_____ 7. allogenic transplant

_____ 8. vesicants

a. small, pinpoint-sized spots of hemorrhage in the skin

b. difficulty walking

c. hair loss

d. dryness of the mouth

e. from a donor

f. skin irritants

g. marked reduction in the number of RBCs, WBCs, and platelets

h. large skin hemorrhage

Multiple Choice

1. Which one of the following statements about childhood cancer is true?

   a. It usually arises from primitive embryonic tissue.
   b. It is usually caused by exposure to carcinogens.
   c. It usually arises from epithelial tissue.
   d. Routine screening is the key to survival.

2. Children receiving chemotherapy often develop thrombocytopenia. Which statement by the child's caregiver indicates that more education on the care of the child is indicated?

   a. My child is at greatest risk for serious life-threatening bacterial infection.
   b. Contact sports should be avoided.
   c. Activities with a risk of injury should be avoided.
   d. I will examine my child for signs of bleeding on a regular basis.

3. Rick is a 4-year-old child who is neutropenic as a result of chemotherapeutic treatment for leukemia. When teaching his parents how to care for Rick at home, the nurse includes which one of the following statements?

   a. Rick will show exaggerated signs of an infection should he develop one. Be on the lookout for high fevers.
   b. Rick has immunity to common childhood illnesses such as chickenpox due to this condition.
   c. Rick should not receive the oral preparation of polio vaccine (OPV) or the measles, mumps, rubella (MMR) vaccine at this time.
   d. Rick is at high risk for uncontrolled bleeding.

4. Which of the following cancer treatment modalities stimulates the immune system to destroy cancer cells and accelerates hematopoiesis?

   a. chemotherapy
   b. radiation therapy
   c. bone marrow transplant
   d. biological response modifiers

5. Pedro, age 8, is receiving antineoplastic drugs IV. He is being discharged to home with an external venous access device (VAD). Which statement by Pedro's caregiver indicates that more teaching is needed?

   a. Frequent flushing of the catheter with a heparinized saline solution is needed to maintain patency.

   b. I will assess the exit site daily for signs of infection such as drainage, redness, or pain.

   c. I will not permit Pedro to bathe or swim while the external VAD is in place.

   d. I can expect to use increasing pressure to flush the catheter as it matures.

6. Which statement about safe handling of chemotherapy by the new nurse indicates that more education is needed?

   a. Further research is needed to determine the implication of human exposure to chemotherapy.

   b. Once the chemotherapeutic agent has passed through the client's body, it is inactivated.

   c. Health care providers should use airflow hoods while mixing chemotherapy.

   d. Nurses can be exposed to chemotherapeutic agents through ingestion.

7. Edward, age 6, has been diagnosed with a brain tumor and is scheduled to receive radiation therapy. Which statement by Edward's father indicates that more teaching is needed?

   a. Radiation therapy is used to deliver a therapeutic dose of ionizing radiation to a tumor with minimum effect to the healthy surrounding tissue.

   b. The actual treatment is quite quick, although it takes about 10 to 15 minutes to prepare, position, and actually deliver the treatment.

   c. Radiation therapy is painful, so Edward will be given medication to relieve the pain while the treatment is going on.

   d. Edward will have changes in the mucosa of his mouth, including dryness.

8. Which statement made by the student nurse regarding interleukins indicates that more education is needed?

   a. They directly kill cancer cells.

   b. Interleukin-11 stimulates proliferation of functioning platelets.

   c. Side effects of treatment may include hypotension.

   d. They are proteins that regulate the intensity and duration of immune responses.

9. Which one of the following statements about acute myelogenous leukemia (AML) is true?

    a. Children with this type of leukemia are at high risk for the development of disseminated intravascular coagulation.

    b. Children with AML have a better prognosis than those children with acute lymphocytic leukemia (ALL).

    c. AML is characterized by the development of neutropenia, thrombocytopenia, and anemia.

    d. There is a higher incidence of central nervous system (CNS) disease at diagnosis with AML than with ALL.

10. Which of the following statements about neuroblstoma made by a new nurse will require the supervising nurse to provide additional education?

    a. The diagnosis of neuroblastoma can conclusively be made when neuroblastoma cells in tissue samples are seen under a microscope.

    b. Clients with neuroblastoma undergo frequent radiologic scans to evaluate efficacy of treatment.

    c. A neuroblastoma is a cancerous tumor in the kidney.

    d. When an individual with neuroblastoma is in remission, the urine will be analyzed to assess for metabolites that are markers of a recurrence.

Multiple Response

1. The nurse is providing a talk to a group of parents whose children have cancer. The children are of various age groups and cancer diagnoses. The topic of hair loss is raised by one of the parents. Which of the following should the nurse include? Select all that apply.

    a. Children less than 5 years of age are not as concerned with hair loss as adolescents are.

    b. Hair loss is permanent in children under 10 because the chemotherapy kills the growth root of the hair shaft.

    c. If the child requests a wig, arrangement for the purchase should be done prior to the actual hair loss.

    d. Children with hair loss should protect their heads from sunburn

    e. Children with hair loss should protect their heads from cold weather.

    f. Wigs are not recommended for children because they are difficult to keep on.

2. When caring for a child undergoing whole-brain radiation, the nurse is aware that which of the following are associated complications of this treatment? Select all that apply.

    a. somnolence syndrome
    b. papilledema
    c. acute renal failure
    d. nausea and vomiting
    e. cardiotoxicity
    f. hepatomegaly

3. Nursing care of the child with a brain tumor includes which of the following interventions? Select all that apply.

    a. seizure precautions preoperatively
    b. careful monitoring of fluid balance
    c. preparation for magnetic resonance imaging as the most common first diagnostic test obtained for suspected brain tumor
    d. ensuring no use of sedation in diagnostic testing
    e. seizure precautions postoperatively
    f. careful monitoring of electrolyte balance

4. Which of the following statements about Hodgkin's disease are true? Select all that apply.

    a. Burkitt's lymphoma is a type of Hodgkin's disease.
    b. The onset of Hodgkin's disease is commonly chronic in nature.
    c. Staging evaluation of Hodgkin's disease includes chest X-ray and CT of chest, abdomen, and pelvis to assess for distant lymph node involvement.
    d. Bleomycin and doxorubicin are two commonly used drugs in the treatment of Hodgkin's disease.
    e. Hodgkin's disease is primarily a disorder of the bone.
    f. Only children over 10 years of age can develop Hodgkin's disease.

5. Which of the following statements about osteogenic sarcoma are true? Select all that apply.

    a. It is a tumor of the ligaments.
    b. Fracture is the usual presenting symptom.
    c. When diagnosed there is always metastasis associated with this type of cancer.
    d. Treatment consists of surgical resection of the affected bone.
    e. Treatment consists of chemotherapy.
    f. Pain at the site of the tumor is the most common presenting symptom.

Critical Thinking/Case Study

Beth, age 14, has been diagnosed with leukemia. She has received standard therapy and is now a candidate for hematopoietic stem cell transplantation. The following interaction occurs with Beth, her mother, and the nurse.

1. Beth's mom asks the nurse what the difference is between the different types of hematopoietic stem cell transplant procedures. How does the nurse respond?

   _____

   _____

   _____

2. Beth asks the nurse to explain to her how they will go about finding someone who can be a donor. Beth does not understand how the tissue between recipient and donor is matched. What does the nurse tell Beth?

   _____

   _____

   _____

3. Beth's mom is very interested in finding out information about the procedure and what to expect. How does the nurse summarize the phases of hematopoietic stem cell transplantation?

   _____

   _____

   _____

4. Beth asks the nurse, "I hear about a lot of people who have transplants and then reject them. What can I do to not reject the tissue I get?" What is the nurse's response?

   _____

   _____

   _____

5. Beth's mom is very hopeful that the transplant will be a success. She asks the nurse, "How can we expect Beth's life to change after the transplant? I know it is going to work and that Beth will be fine. What will we need to do after she comes home from the transplant?" Provide the nurse's response.

_____

_____

_____

CHAPTER 30

Integumentary Alterations

True or False

1. The skin and its appendages comprise one of the largest single organs of the body.

   ❑ True   ❑ False

2. The skin plays a vital role in the absorption of ultraviolet light and for the conversion of substances to vitamin C.

   ❑ True   ❑ False

3. The pH of a newborn's skin is relatively alkaline during the first week of life, which renders the infant more susceptible to infection.

   ❑ True   ❑ False

4. Topical medications should be avoided in infants less than 6 months of age.

   ❑ True   ❑ False

5. Dermatophytes are a group of closely related fungi that invade keratonized tissue.

   ❑ True   ❑ False

6. Griseofulvin is the agent most commonly used to treat tinea capitis.

   ❑ True   ❑ False

7. When used to treat herpes simplex 1 infections, acyclovir (Zovirax) breaks down the cell wall of the virus, causing cell death.

   ❑ True   ❑ False

8. Spread of lice is caused by their flying or jumping from individual to individual.

   ❑ True   ❑ False

9. Occlusive agents such as petroleum jelly and olive oil are recommended agents to use in the treatment of pediculosis.

   ❑ True   ❑ False

10. Because of the long incubation period associated with scabies, all household members and close physical contacts should be treated prophylactically.

    ❑ True   ❑ False

11. Current practice for atopic dermatitis includes short daily baths followed by patting the skin dry and the immediate application of an emollient.

    ❑ True   ❑ False

12. Recommended treatment of diaper dermatitis includes changing the diaper every 2-4 hours with application of topical steroid with every diaper change.

    ❑ True   ❑ False

13. Topical corticosteroids are the mainstay of therapy for atopic dermatitis.

    ❑ True   ❑ False

14. Infection rates are significantly greater following dog bites than cat bites.

    ❑ True   ❑ False

15. The diagnosis of rabies is confirmed by demonstration of virus-specific fluorescent antigen in the tissue of the liver.

    ❑ True   ❑ False

16. Tanning is a reparative response and indicates that the skin has been damaged.

    ❑ True   ❑ False

17. If a child has sustained a brown recluse spider bite, the immediate treatment consists of rest, ice, and elevation.

    ❑ True   ❑ False

18. Thrush usually responds quickly to administration of topical corticosteroids.

    ❑ True   ❑ False

19. Pulse dosing involves switching between periods when medications are administered followed by drug-free intervals.

    ❑ True   ❑ False

20. Variations in hair texture and curl of African Americans may contribute to the increased incidence of pediculosis observed in this population.

    ❑ True   ❑ False

Fill in the Blank

1. The metabolic functions of the skin include _____ and _____.

2. _____ is a highly contagious superficial bacterial skin infection.

3. The classic symptoms of cellulitis are those of an acute inflammatory process, _____, _____, _____, and _____.

4. Candidiasis also may present as _____, an erythematous skin eruption occurring on apposed skin surfaces.

5. The tinea infections include _____ (head ringworm), _____ (body ringworm), _____ (athlete's foot), _____ (jock itch), and _____ or _____ (nail fungus).

6. An antifungal medication that may offer a more definitive cure with a shorter duration of treatment is _____.

7. After an animal bite, tetanus immunizations should be given to those individuals who have not been immunized for tetanus previously and to those who have not had a tetanus immunization in the past _____ years.

8. The initial drug of choice in the event of an anaphylactic reaction is subcutaneous _____.

9. A _____ is a painful, firm, walled-off mass of granulation tissue and pus. It is more commonly known as an abscess or a boil.

10. The characteristic black color of blackheads is not from dirt, but occurs as a consequence of oxidation of _____.

11. _____ is the first agent of a new class of topical antibiotics used to treat mupirocin resistant strains of s. aureus.

Matching

_____ 1. hyphae

_____ 2. desquamation

_____ 3. cellulitis

_____ 4. mycosis

_____ 5. impetigo

_____ 6. fomites

_____ 7. alopecia

_____ 8. lichenification

_____ 9. thrush

_____ 10. verrucae

_____ 11. spongiosis

_____ 12. pediculosis

a. fungal infection

b. warts

c. bald spots

d. creamy-white plaques on the buccal mucosa and lateral borders of the tongue

e. thickening of the skin with exaggeration of its normal markings

f. shedding of the outer layer of the epidermis

g. lice

h. branching outgrowths of a fungus that invades the tissue and establishes an infection

i. inanimate objects on which disease-causing organisms may be conveyed

j. honey-colored crusts

k. bacterial infection of the dermis and subcutaneous tissue

l. inflammation of the skin's spongy layer

Multiple Choice

1. Which statement by a caregiver of a child with impetigo indicates that more teaching is needed?

    a. Impetigo is highly contagious.
    b. Other individuals living in our home, especially children, should be examined for signs of infection.
    c. Uncomplicated lesions generally heal without scarring.
    d. I will keep my child out of school until the lesions are completely gone and the skin resumes a normal appearance.

2. Nathan, age 7 weeks, has been diagnosed with thrush. Which one of the following statements should the nurse include in teaching Nathan's caregivers how to care for this condition?

   a. If you are breastfeeding, you must switch to bottles for the infection to clear up.
   b. Administer the medication to Nathan before his feedings.
   c. Use a Toothette to swab the medication on the mucosal surfaces of the mouth.
   d. Expect to see a whitish discharge from the infected area indicating resolution of the problem.

3. The school nurse is asked to evaluate a child with a rash. The nurse observes an annular lesion with an erythematous border. The nurse suspects this to most likely be:

   a. impetigo
   b. tinea corporis
   c. chicken pox
   d. psoriasis

4. Which of the following statements about scabies is true?

   a. Infants are the age group most commonly affected by this condition.
   b. The medication for treatment should be quickly applied and immediately washed off.
   c. Itching is most intense during the day.
   d. The most characteristic manifestation is a burrow mark of the skin.

5. Justin, age 3 months, has diaper dermatitis. His caregiver asks the nurse what he should use to clean Justin's skin when changing his diaper. The best response by the nurse is:

   a. mild soap and water
   b. baby wipes
   c. lotions
   d. antibiotic ointment

6. Which medication used in the management of acne vulgaris has a side effect of elevated triglyceride levels?

   a. isotretinoin (Accutane)
   b. tretinoin (Retin-a)
   c. erythromycin
   d. topical benzoyl peroxide

7. Which of the following statements about acne is true?

   a. It is caused by dirt left on the face.

   b. Keeping hair clean and off the forehead tends to lessen the severity of the lesions.

   c. Foods high in caffeine have been demonstrated to increase the occurrence of acne.

   d. Aggressive washing of the face has been shown to be the best treatment for acne.

8. An 8-year-old child has been taught how to avoid being bitten by a dog. Which statement by the child indicates that more teaching is needed?

   a. If an unfamiliar dog approaches me, I will stay still like a tree.

   b. I will look at dogs in their eyes when I talk to them.

   c. I will not pet a dog without allowing it to see and sniff me first.

   d. If I get knocked over by a dog, I will roll into a ball and lie still.

9. Which statement by a 14-year-old girl receiving isotretinoin (Accutane) indicates that more teaching is indicated?

   a. If I were to become pregnant the medication could have severe effects on my baby.

   b. Use of this medication is reserved for people with severe inflammatory acne who have not responded to standard therapies.

   c. I will need to have my blood checked to monitor for side effects of this medication.

   d. If this medication does not work within two weeks, I will not be able to ever receive it again.

10. A child has been diagnosed with scabies. Which statement by the caregiver indicates that more teaching is needed?

    a. Multiple applications of the scabicide are always necessary for effectiveness to be obtained.

    b. The scabicide should be applied to all areas of the body with particular attention given to the skin folds, fingernails, toenails, scalp, and posterior auricular areas.

    c. Topical lubricants such as fragrance-free lotions and creams often are sufficient to manage pruritus following treatment.

    d. Children may return to school or day care 24 hours after the completion of treatment for scabies.

Multiple Response

1. Which of the following statements about Mongolian spots are true? Select all that apply.

   a. They most commonly occur with light-skinned infants.

   b. They are often misdiagnosed as bruises commonly found in child abuse.

   c. They are most commonly found over the lumbosacral area of the infant.

   d. They are a bluish-black hyperpigmentation of the skin.

   e. They become darker as the child gets older.

   f. They occur in 100% of Asian individuals.

2. Rahema, age 2, has been diagnosed with impetigo. The nurse will perform which of the following interventions? Select all that apply.

   a. gentle washing of the skin

   b. use of gloves during care

   c. administration of prescribed antiviral creams

   d. assessment for lymphadenopathy

   e. use of mittens to prevent scratching

   f. gentle removal of crusts

3. Mabel, age 5 months, has been diagnosed with a severe case of diaper rash. Her care-giver has been advised to use ointments and barrier creams to treat the rash. Which of the following procedures should be followed when applying the ointments and barrier creams to Mabel's diaper rash? Select all that apply.

   a. Use prescribed steroid products for no more than two weeks.

   b. Apply the ointments and barrier creams in a thick layer.

   c. When the diaper is soiled, wipe the top layer of the ointment or barrier cream away.

   d. Use sterile technique when applying the ointments and barrier creams.

   e. Change Mabel's diaper at least every 2 to 4 hours.

   f. Use an alcohol-based product to remove the barrier creams from Mabel's skin.

4. After sustaining a bee sting, a child experiences an anaphylactic reaction. Which of the following are manifestations of anaphylaxis? Select all that apply.

   a. marked drowsiness and lethargy

   b. abdominal cramping

   c. shortness of breath

   d. nausea

   e. wheezing

   f. edema of the tongue

Critical Thinking/Case Study

A local community day care center has had an outbreak of pediculosis capitis. Children were treated, but an almost immediate reinfestation has occurred. A nurse from the community health department has been asked to assess the situation and provide assistance in eradicating this problem.

1. What does the nurse need to know about the incidence and etiology of pediculosis capitis?

   _____

   _____

   _____

2. The staff at the day care center ask the nurse how the lice are spread. What would be the best response by the nurse?

   _____

   _____

   _____

3. With so many children in the day care center and so many caregivers concerned about the outbreak, what information should the nurse give these individuals about the clinical manifestation of pediculosis capitis?

   _____

   _____

   _____

4. What pharmacologic treatment is recommended for pediculosis capitis?

_____

_____

_____

5. What environmental measures need to be taken by the day care and in the homes of infested children?

_____

_____

_____

6. What teaching can be included by the nurse to reduce the chance of recurrence of this problem in the future?

_____

_____

_____

CHAPTER 31

Sensory Alterations

True or False

1. The link between hearing loss in children and poor communication has been well documented.

   ❑ True   ❑ False

2. The first three to four years of childhood are the most important for speech and language development.

   ❑ True   ❑ False

3. The earlier correction of language disorders is accomplished, the less learning delay will occur.

   ❑ True   ❑ False

4. To avoid confusion and difficulties in language development, children should be taught one language at a time.

   ❑ True   ❑ False

5. The noise level in neonatal intensive care units is producing hearing loss in newborns, especially in premature low birth-weight babies.

   ❑ True   ❑ False

6. Sensorineural hearing loss can be improved with use of a hearing aid to amplify sound.

   ❑ True   ❑ False

7. Permanent eye color of a baby is established at 6 months of age.

   ❑ True   ❑ False

8. Refractive disorders are the most common type of visual disorders in children.

   ❑ True   ❑ False

9. Correction of strabismus must occur before 2 years of age or correction of the problem will not be possible.

   ❑ True   ❑ False

10. Visual acuity can only be assessed indirectly in children less than 3 years of age.

   ❑ True   ❑ False

11. A 5-year-old with normal language development should be able to easily communicate and carry on a conversation with an adult.

   ❑ True   ❑ False

12. When interventions are begun for an infant with a hearing loss prior to 6 months of age, the infant will most likely experience age-appropriate social, emotional, and communication skills.

   ❑ True   ❑ False

13. Development of the eye is not complete at birth.

   ❑ True   ❑ False

Fill in the Blank

1. _____ involves the physical production of sound using the oral mechanism.

2. _____ is a speech impairment in which an individual involuntarily repeats a sound or word, resulting in loss of speech fluency.

3. The primary nursing responsibilities when caring for children with communication impairments are _____ and _____.

4. _____ is a temporary or permanent hearing deficit resulting from any condition, such as fluids, that affects the progress of sound into the ear canal or across the middle ear system. _____ results from damage or malformation of the middle ear and/or auditory nerve.

5. Loudness is described in terms of _____ units, and frequency is described in terms of _____ units.

6. _____ are devices that present acoustic information decoded tactually on the skin's surface for the purpose of speech reception.

7. _____ is a method of communication that uses eight configurations and four positions of the hand to supplement lip reading when words look alike when formed by the lips.

8. _____ occurs when there is uneven curvature of the cornea or lens, preventing light rays from focusing correctly on the retina.

9. _____ is a condition in which the visual lines of each eye do not simultaneously focus on the same object in space due to a lack of muscle coordination, resulting in a crossed-eye appearance.

10. _____ is a reduction or loss of vision in one eye unrelated to an organic cause.

11. Visual acuity assessment is not possible in children under _____ years of age.

Matching

_____ 1. conductive hearing loss

_____ 2. epiphoria

_____ 3. myopia

_____ 4. esotropia

_____ 5. binocularity

_____ 6. exotropia

_____ 7. hyperopia

_____ 8. pitch

_____ 9. conjunctivitis

_____ 10. loudness

_____ 11. Ishihara

_____ 12. sensorineural hearing loss

_____ 13. hyphema

_____ 14. buphthalmos

_____ 15.

_____ 16. astigmatism

_____ 17. amblyopia

a. eyes turn away from midline

b. nearsightedness

c. tearing

d. intensity

e. damage or malformation of the middle ear

f. eyes turn toward midline

g. frequency

h. pink eye

i. hemorrhage of the anterior chamber of the eye

j. fixation of two ocular images into one cerebral picture

k. farsightedness

l. lack of muscle coordination of the eye

m. blurred vision

n. enlarged eyeball

o. affects the progression of sound into the ear canal or across the middle ear system

p. loss of vision of one eye unrelated to organic causes

q. color plates

Multiple Choice

1. The nurse is assessing a 4-year-old child's language development. Which of the following terms refers to the ordering or arrangement of words to communicate an idea?

   a. articulation
   b. semantics
   c. syntax
   d. fluency

2. Ms. W asks the nurse what is the most effective way to deal with her 5-year-old daughter who stutters. The most appropriate response by the nurse would be:

   a. Your daughter will outgrow stuttering by the time she is 8.
   b. Decreasing stress is most helpful in decreasing stuttering.
   c. Do not make eye contact with your daughter when she stutters.
   d. Use a fast rate of speech when talking to your daughter.

3. The nurse assesses which of the following children as most likely to have a speech and language disorder?

   a. a 6-month-old who turns eyes and head to sound
   b. a 2-year-old who is not talking at all
   c. a 3-year-old with noticeably impaired sentence structure
   d. a 1-year-old who does not respond to directions appropriately

4. Robbie, a 6-year-old boy, has been recently diagnosed as being color blind. Which statement by his mother indicates that more teaching is needed?

   a. Colorblindness occurs more frequently in males than females.
   b. Robbie has difficulty distinguishing red from green colors.
   c. Robbie has difficulty distinguishing blue from yellow colors.
   d. The condition can be cured with the use of Ishihara lenses.

5. The nurse would expect to see which behavior as representative of a milestone of normal hearing development for a 5-month-old?

   a. dances and makes sounds to music
   b. smiles when spoken to
   c. looks at an object or picture when someone speaks about it
   d. stops for a minute on hearing "no-no"

6. When communicating with a hearing impaired child, the nurse will avoid doing which of the following?

    a. encouraging use of a hearing aid

    b. eliminating background noise

    c. speaking with a loud volume

    d. avoiding restraining the child's hands

7. Which statement about the use of contact lenses in an adolescent indicates that more teaching is needed?

    a. Contact lenses improve body image.

    b. Contact lenses are not as safe as glasses for children who are engaged in active sports.

    c. Care and cleaning directions must be followed explicitly in order to avoid complications such as corneal damage.

    d. Allergic reaction to the cleaning solution can include itching and burning of the eyes.

8. Which of the following treatment modalities for care of a child with viral conjunctivitis will the nurse question?

    a. cold compress to the eye

    b. acetaminophen

    c. reduction of light

    d. antibacterials

9. Which of the following assessment findings in a newborn indicate potential visual loss?

    a. squinting

    b. rubbing eyes

    c. corneal clouding

    d. clear lens

10. When caring for a child who has sustained a chemical burn to the eye, which action by the new nurse requires the supervising nurse to intervene? The new nurse:

    a. flushes the eye from the outer to inner canthus

    b. uses pH paper to determine acidity of the fluid of the eye

    c. administers cycloleptic drugs

    d. administers antibiotics

Multiple Response

1. When communicating with a child who stutters, it is most effective for the nurse to do which of the following? Select all that apply.

   a. Ask the child to speed up his or her rate of speech.
   b. Positively reinforce periods of fluent speech.
   c. Ask open-ended questions.
   d. Maintain eye contact.
   e. Avoid appearing hurried.
   f. Speak to the child in a loud voice.

2. The nurse is teaching the parents of Amy, age 18 months, how to care for her hearing aid. Which of the following will the nurse include? Select all that apply.

   a. Hearing aids amplify the speaker's voice, which can be annoying and confusing to a child.
   b. Heat will damage the hearing aid.
   c. The hearing aid will need to be replaced on a yearly basis.
   d. The ear mold is the only part that can be cleaned with pipe cleaners or toothbrushes.
   e. Hearing aids do not amplify background noise.
   f. Moisture will not damage a hearing aid.

3. Jayne is born with a cataract in her right eye. Her mother asks the nurse, "How can this possibly happen to my baby? Old people get cataracts. What can you tell me about cataracts and babies?" How should the nurse reply? Select all that apply.

   a. The cataract in your baby will be treated with medicine and dissolve within the first month of life.
   b. Jayne will need to wear a corrective lens or contact lens to focus light on the retina.
   c. Treatment must take place before 8 weeks of age to prevent an irreversible lack of vision development.
   d. Early identification is essential to prevent the suppression of development of the visual cortex in the brain.
   e. Babies born with cataracts have diabetes mellitus.
   f. Your baby will be blind in the eye that has the cataract.

4. The nurse is at the scene of an accident where an 11-year-old boy has sustained an injury to the face and has an object in his eye. The nurse will perform which of the following activities? Select all that apply.

   a. Cover the uninjured eye.
   b. Remove the object from the eye.
   c. Secure the object with tape to prevent movement.
   d. Transport the child to the emergency department.
   e. Assess movement in the uninjured eye.
   f. Flush the injured eye with copious amounts of tap water.

Critical Thinking/Case Study

A nurse has been asked to speak to a group of adults from the community for several evenings on safety issues with children. The topic for this evening's talk is eye trauma, which is a frequent occurrence in the pediatric population.

1. What information should the nurse relay to the audience about the incidence and etiology of eye trauma?

   _____
   _____
   _____

2. What are the differences between penetrating and nonpenetrating eye trauma?

   _____
   _____
   _____

3. What are some ways to prevent eye trauma?

   _____
   _____
   _____

4. What is part of emergency treatment for eye trauma?

_____

_____

_____

5. How can the incidence of eye injuries in sports be decreased?

_____

_____

_____

6. What effect does exposure to ultraviolet rays from the sun have on the eyes?

_____

_____

_____

7. How can this damage be prevented?

_____

_____

_____

CHAPTER 32

Neurological Alterations

True or False

1. An infant is better able to accommodate to rising intracranial pressure than an older child.

   ❑ True ❑ False

2. Children are able to recover more quickly and completely than adults after neurologic injury.

   ❑ True ❑ False

3. At the first indication of a child having a seizure, a tongue blade should be placed in the child's mouth.

   ❑ True ❑ False

4. Morphine sulfate is the drug of choice for a child in status epilepticus.

   ❑ True ❑ False

5. The signs and symptoms of hydrocephalus are generally due to an increase in size of the ventricles.

   ❑ True ❑ False

6. The typical treatment for hydrocephalus is surgical intervention.

   ❑ True ❑ False

7. Infection is the most serious complication associated with ventriculoperitoneal shunt placement.

   ❑ True ❑ False

8. Pressure ulcer development is the most common complication associated with spina bifida.

   ❑ True ❑ False

9. Infants with spina bifida not yet surgically corrected should be placed in the supine position.

   ❑ True   ❑ False

10. Hypothermia is a common manifestation of children with meningitis.

    ❑ True   ❑ False

11. Family members and others who come into close contact with children who have meningococcemia must be treated prophylactically with rifampin.

    ❑ True   ❑ False

12. Bacterial meningitis is generally considered a more benign disease than viral meningitis, as most children recover quickly and without incident.

    ❑ True   ❑ False

13. Steroids are one of the primary drugs indicated in the acute treatment of children with head trauma.

    ❑ True   ❑ False

14. The American Academy of Pediatrics states that children under the age of 3 years are too young to learn to swim.

    ❑ True   ❑ False

15. Cold-water near-drowning victims have a better chance of recovery than victims of warm-water near drowning.

    ❑ True   ❑ False

Fill in the Blank

1. _____ or flexor posturing is associated with bilateral cerebral hemisphere injury, while _____ or rigid extensor posturing is secondary to trauma to the midbrain or pons.

2. Seizures are the result of a spontaneous electrical discharge of hyperexcited brain cells in an area called the _____.

3. _____ is a prolonged seizure or series of convulsions where loss of consciousness occurs for at least 30 minutes. _____ seizures last more than 60 minutes, and _____ refers to a chronic seizure disorder that is often associated with central nervous system pathology.

4. _____ are manifested as tonic/clonic movements of the face with increased salivation and arrested speech that commonly occur during sleep, while _____ are motor episodes, beginning with tonic contractions of either the fingers of one hand, toes of one foot, or one side of the face, that "march" up adjacent muscles of the affected extremity or side of the body.

5. The _____ diet has gained popularity in treating absence, akinetic, and myoclonic seizures.

6. Infants with hydrocephalus exhibit a positive _____, or a hollow or "cracked-pot" sound, produced on percussion of the skull.

7. Low levels of _____ in mothers have been associated with spina bifida in their children.

8. A _____ is a saclike extrusion through the spinal cord containing the meninges, cerebrospinal fluid, and a portion of the spinal cord and/or nerve roots. A _____ is a saclike herniation through the bony malformation of the spine containing the meninges and cerebrospinal fluid.

9. Amniocentesis may be used to diagnose some neural tube defects prenatally. An increase in _____ in the amniotic fluid indicates the presence of meningomyelocele.

10. If a child complains of a migraine-like headache and has a seizure, there should be high suspicion of a(n) _____.

11. A child with nuchal rigidity will assume a(n) _____ position whereby the head and neck are hyperextended.

12. _____ is evoked when a child is supine and the head is flexed forward with the child automatically flexing the hips and knees. _____ is tested by having the child lie supine with hips flexed; if meningitis is present, the child will either resist the examiner's attempts to extend the leg or complain about pain on extension.

13. _____ is the most serious form of alteration in level of consciousness.

14. _____ is the first drug that is most often administered for the child experiencing a seizure.

Matching

_____ 1. craniostenosis

_____ 2. encephalocele

_____ 3. lordosis

_____ 4. Reye's syndrome

_____ 5. rhizotomy

_____ 6. rachischisis

_____ 7. encephalocele

_____ 8. cranioschisis

_____ 9. kyphosis

_____ 10. cerebral palsy

_____ 11. decorticate

_____ 12. Dandy-Walker syndrome

_____ 13. dura mater

_____ 14. confusion

_____ 15. seizures

_____ 16. stupor

_____ 17. hydrocephalus

a. acute life-threatening encephalopathy with accompanying microvascular fatty deposits in the liver and kidney

b. fissure in the vertebral column, exposing the meninges and spinal cord

c. malformation in which the brain is totally exposed or herniated through a defect in the skull

d. premature closure of the cranial sutures

e. a protrusion of the brain and meninges into a fluid-filled sac through a defect in the skull

f. forward curvature of the spine

g. abnormal curvature of the thoracic spine

h. small section of the spinal cord is cut

i. nonprogressive motor dysfunction due to damage in the motor areas of the brain

j. defect in the skull through which neural tissue protrudes

k. obstruction in the foramina of Luschka and Magendie

l. excessive amount of cerebrospinal fluid within the cerebral ventricles

m. membrane attached to the brain tissue itself

n. unresponsive state

o. flexor posturing

p. herniation of the cerebellum, medulla, pons, and fourth ventricle into the cervical canal through an enlarged foramen magnum

q. membrane covering the brain

_____ 18. decerebrate

_____ 19. Arnold-Chiari malformation

_____ 20. meninges

_____ 21. coma

_____ 22. delirium

_____ 23. spina bifida

_____ 24. pia mater

r. disoriented to time, place, and person

s. anxiety, fear, and agitation are seen

t. no response to intense painful stimuli

u. rigid extensor posturing

v. membrane that adheres to the inner surface of the skull

w. episodic, stereotypic behavioral syndromes

x. due to failure of the neural tube to close completely or a fissure resulting from increased cerebrospinal fluid pressure

Multiple Choice

1. Fever is a common etiology for which type of seizure?

    a. complex

    b. myoclonic

    c. tonic/clonic

    d. absence

2. Which statement by the caregiver of a child with simple partial seizures indicates that more teaching is needed?

    a. My child will only experience these seizures for the first year of life.

    b. There is no aura associated with these episodes.

    c. My child generally will not lose consciousness with this type of seizure.

    d. The symptoms seen are most often motor or sensory in nature.

3. When working with a child who experiences generalized seizures, the nurse is aware of the fact that these types of seizures:

    a. are accompanied by an aura

    b. are always associated with loss of consciousness

    c. arise from both cerebral hemispheres

    d. last from several seconds to hours

4. Which statement about febrile seizures is true?

   a. They are a type of tonic/clonic seizure.

   b. They usually occur in children who are 5 to 10 years of age.

   c. They can occur at a temperature of 37.8°C (100°F).

   d. An aura that lasts for less than 15 minutes frequently occurs.

5. A new nurse is caring for an 11-year-old child with an external ventricular drain. Which statement by the new nurse indicates that more training is needed? The new nurse identifies signs of overdraining of the external ventricular drain as causing:

   a. seizures

   b. change in blood pressure

   c. severe headache

   d. increased heart rate

6. Jorge, age 2 months, has had a ventriculoperitoneal shunt placed for hydrocephalus. The nurse caring for him in the postoperative period should place him in which position?

   a. flat on the unoperated side

   b. flat on the operated side

   c. head elevated 90 degrees on the unoperated side

   d. head elevated 90 degrees on the operated side

7. Which statement by the new nurse indicates more teaching is needed? When caring for a child who is chemically paralyzed indications of pain include:

   a. bradycardia

   b. pallor

   c. increased blood pressure

   d. tears

8. The nurse determines which one of the following children as a possible candidate for lumbar puncture?

   a. Helena, age 3, exhibiting signs and symptoms of Cushing's triad

   b. Morgan, age 8, who has disseminated intravascular coagulation

   c. Nathan, age 2, with fever of unknown origin

   d. Shaquile, age 7, who sustained an injury to the face after accidentally being hit with a baseball bat while playing with his friends

9. When teaching caregivers to avoid use of over-the-counter medications that contain aspirin, the nurse identifies which one of the following medications as not containing aspirin?

    a. Advil

    b. Pepto-Bismol

    c. Excedrin

    d. Alka-Seltzer

10. Which of the following statements about subdural hemorrhages in children is true?

    a. They result from damage to cerebral arteries.

    b. They may occur with and without skull fracture.

    c. Signs and symptoms occur immediately at all times and result in quick deterioration of the client status.

    d. Occurrence in children is very rare.

11. Devan, age 8, who was not wearing a helmet, fell off a scooter and sustained a head injury. While caring for Devan, the student nurse incorrectly identifies which of the following as a sign or symptom of increased intracranial pressure?

    a. increased systolic pressure

    b. widened pulse pressure

    c. hypotension

    d. bradycardia

12. A spinal cord lesion at which level is most likely to cause paraplegia?

    a. C-5

    b. C-6

    c. C-7

    d. T-1

13. Alex, age 7, has cerebral palsy. He exhibits constant involuntary writhing motions that affect his entire body. The nurse would best describe this behavior exhibited by Alex as:

    a. ataxia

    b. hypotonia

    c. athetosis

    d. hypertonia

14. A nurse arrives at a scene where a 2-year-old child has just fallen down a flight of stairs. The child is lying at the bottom of the stairs. He has a glazed look on his face. The nurse suspects spinal cord injury. No apparent bleeding is noted. After determining that the child has a patent airway and is breathing, the nurse should do which of the following?

   a. Assist the child to a sitting position.
   b. Ask the child to flex and extend all extremities.
   c. Maintain the child in the position in which he or she was found, preventing any movement.
   d. Instruct the caregiver to pick the child up to provide comfort.

15. A nurse practicing in a clinic for children with cerebral palsy performs an assessment on a child and finds the child to have irregularity in muscle action and coordination with intention tremors. The child also has a wide-based gait. The nurse would describe these characteristics as which type of cerebral palsy?

   a. hypotonia
   b. hypertonia
   c. athetosis
   d. ataxia

Multiple Response

1. Jamie, age 4, was not wearing a helmet when he fell off his bicycle, and he sustained a head injury. He is being observed in the pediatric intensive care unit. Which of the following are consistent with Cushing's triad? Select all that apply.

   a. increased systolic blood pressure
   b. bradycardia
   c. wide pulse pressure
   d. vomiting
   e. nausea
   f. dilated pupils

2. Which of the following are factors predisposing young children to alterations in neurologic function? Select all that apply.

    a. high levels of serotonin
    b. very vascular brain prone to hemorrhage
    c. dura that can easily peel from the inner surface of the skull
    d. large subarachnoid space
    e. fragile neurons
    f. immature immune system

3. Amy, age 12, was rock climbing with her family when a belt snapped and she fell, sustaining a spinal cord injury at C-7. Upon assessment of Amy in the emergency department, which of the following indicate that Amy is in spinal shock? Select all that apply.

    a. spastic extremities
    b. loss of deep tendon reflexes
    c. no sensory response
    d. atonic bladder
    e. tachycardia
    f. hypertension

4. When caring for a child with spinal cord injury, the nurse is aware of the need to assess for the development of autonomic dysreflexia. Which of the following are clinical manifestations of autonomic dysreflexia? Select all that apply.

    a. perfuse perspiration above the level of the injury
    b. headache
    c. bradycardia
    d. hypotension
    e. urticaria
    f. incontinence

5. Which of the following statements about Ketogenic diet does the nurse identify as true? Select all that apply.

    a. the diet is high in protein
    b. the diet is low in carbohydrates
    c. fat is used as fuel
    d. alkalosis is a common complication
    e. hyperglycemia is a common complication
    f. renal stones are a frequent complication

Critical Thinking/Case Study

A 2-year-old child has just been diagnosed with cerebral palsy. Her caregivers are very concerned. Although the child has not been meeting developmental milestones appropriate for her developmental level at each visit to the primary care provider, the caregivers are shocked that something could be wrong with their child now that a diagnosis has been made. An interaction takes place between the caregivers and the nurse at the primary care office. How could the nurse best respond to the following questions asked by the caregivers?

1. Why wasn't this problem picked up when she was born? We were told that our baby was fine! Something could have been done all this time if we knew something was wrong, isn't that so?

   _____

   _____

   _____

2. I feel so guilty that this happened! What did I do to cause this to occur to my baby?

   _____

   _____

   _____

3. Why did it take so long for them to tell us that something was wrong with our baby?

   _____

   _____

   _____

4. Well, now that we know there is something wrong, what can be done to correct the problem? I want the best specialist to see my child.

   _____

   _____

   _____

5. We have no family in the area, and we have a 3-year-old and a 5-year-old at home. How are we ever going to handle this? Can you help us?

_____

_____

_____

Cognitive Alterations

True or False

1. Most children with profound retardation also have an identified neurological condition causing their retardation.

   ❏ True   ❏ False

2. Many caregivers react with significant grief when they learn that their child is mentally retarded.

   ❏ True   ❏ False

3. Nurses and physicians should make the final decision regarding placement of a child with mental retardation.

   ❏ True   ❏ False

4. Children with Down syndrome often develop Alzheimer's disease after the age of 30.

   ❏ True   ❏ False

5. All children with autism are mentally retarded.

   ❏ True   ❏ False

6. Fragile X syndrome is the most commonly inherited cause of mental retardation.

   ❏ True   ❏ False

7. Definitive prenatal prediction of Down syndrome involves amniocentesis or chorionic villus sampling.

   ❏ True   ❏ False

8. Autism is a genetic developmental disorder, characterized by extreme difficulty communicating with and relating to the environment.

   ❏ True   ❏ False

9. There is no set standard treatment for mental retardation.

   ❑ True   ❑ False

10. Autism is the most widely recognized of the autistic spectrum disorders.

   ❑ True   ❑ False

Fill in the Blank

1. _____ is defined as significantly subaverage general intellectual functioning manifested before age 18, with limited adaptive skills in at least two or more areas of functioning, including communication, self-care, social skills, community use, self-direction, health and safety, academics, and work.

2. The ability of neural cells in a certain area of the brain to assume the functions of a different area, or the ability of the brain to act as a computer does in rerouting signals around a nonfunctioning piece of circuitry, is referred to as _____.

3. The grieving process is composed of six principal states: _____, _____, _____, _____, _____, and _____.

4. Definitive diagnosis of Down syndrome is based on _____, or identification of the chromosomes' appearance, performed by growing out cells from a blood or tissue sample, staining them during the metaphase stage of replication, and scanning them with a microscope.

5. Medically, children with fragile X syndrome are prone to _____ from early childhood and are also at risk for _____ and for _____.

6. According to the American Academy of Pediatrics Committee on Children with Disabilities, the hallmark for autistic disorder is _____.

7. Characteristic features seen in the infant with fetal alcohol syndrome include prenatal and/or postnatal growth retardation, central nervous system neurodevelopmental abnormalities of varying severity, facial dysmorphology, and other abnormalities such as _____, _____, _____, and _____.

8. The autistic spectrum disorders consist of _____, _____, _____, _____, and_____.

Matching

_____ 1. Fragile X syndrome

_____ 2. mosaicism

_____ 3. karyotyping

_____ 4. plasticity

_____ 5. amniocentesis

_____ 6. syndrome

_____ 7. echolalia

_____ 8. atlantoaxial deformity

a. repeating of the last word or words heard

b. identification of chromosome appearance

c. named condition characterized by a group of findings or attributes

d. two different cell lines in an individual or organism

e. common inherited cause of mental retardation

f. instability of the upper cervical spine

g. ability of nerve cells in certain areas of the brain to assume the function of a different area

h. chorionic villus sampling

Multiple Choice

1. Children with Down syndrome are most likely to have defects of which organ?

    a. liver
    b. heart
    c. pancreas
    d. kidney

2. When planning to work with a 5-year-old child who is autistic, the nurse should do which of the following?

    a. Enlist the help of several people at one time to teach the child.
    b. Use music and background sounds to help the child concentrate on the tasks at hand.
    c. Let the child determine the routine to follow.
    d. Provide a highly structured environment with as much one-on-one instruction as possible.

3. The first stage of grief experienced by caregivers of a child newly diagnosed with mental retardation is:

   a. denial

   b. anxiety

   c. depression

   d. anger

4. Which of the following is an expected clinical manifestation of the child with autism?

   a. rigid body form

   b. staring constant eye contact when communicating

   c. hyperresponsiveness to auditory stimuli

   d. altered response to pain

5. A child with fetal alcohol syndrome will most likely manifest:

   a. ptosis

   b. fat upper lip

   c. large eyes

   d. maxillary hyperplasia

Multiple Response

1. When assessing an infant, which of the following are indicative of mental retardation? Select all that apply.

   a. diminished spontaneous activity

   b. poor eye contact during feeding

   c. increased alertness to voices or movements

   d. nonresponsiveness to contact

   e. Apgar score of 7

   f. meconium ileus

2. Clinical manifestations associated with Down syndrome include which of the following? Select all that apply.

   a. hypertonic musculature

   b. a large tongue in a small mouth

   c. epicanthic folds

   d. small nose

   e. depressed nasal bridge

   f. low-set ears

3. A boy with fragile X syndrome would most likely have which of the following characteristics? Select all that apply.

   a. broad, heavy build

   b. large ears

   c. velvet-like skin

   d. large testes

   e. cupping of the ears

   f. close-set wide-open eyes

Critical Thinking/Case Study

Jill, age 3, has just been diagnosed with autism. Her caregivers are in shock. They cannot believe there could be anything wrong with their little girl. The caregivers ask the nurse the following questions. How could the nurse best respond?

1. How can this be? When Jill was born, the doctors told us that she was healthy. There must be some kind of mistake!

   _____

   _____

   _____

2. We adopted Jill when she was 1 month old. Her biological mother must have abused her in the time she had Jill. I have heard that poor mothering skills are responsible for autism.

   _____

   _____

   _____

3. Do you think it was from the immunizations we let Jill have? I knew it, those immuniza-
    tions are nothing but trouble. None of those diseases are around anyway. Why did I let
    them hurt my baby?

    _____

    _____

    _____

4. I don't think Jill loves me anymore. I see all the other children her age in our play group
    hug and kiss their mommies. Why doesn't she love me? Am I a bad mother?

    _____

    _____

    _____

5. There must be a cure for this problem. By gosh, it is the 21st century. We will go any-
    where and do anything to help our baby. Where can we go for a cure?

    _____

    _____

    _____

CHAPTER 34

Musculoskeletal Alterations

True or False

1. Bone is unique as a tissue and an organ because it is a rigid and variable structure, and it can heal and replace itself with normal tissue without scarring.

   ❏ True   ❏ False

2. Maturation and bone shaping continues until 16 years of age.

   ❏ True   ❏ False

3. School-aged children are most at risk for musculoskeletal injury when compared to other age groups of children.

   ❏ True   ❏ False

4. In young children, sprains and strains are very uncommon because the growth plates, or physes, are weaker than the ligaments and will usually separate before a ligament will tear.

   ❏ True   ❏ False

5. With Buck's extension traction, a boot or circular wrap is applied to the skin.

   ❏ True   ❏ False

6. Musculoskeletal pain associated with soft tissue damage fractures, muscle spasms, surgical procedures, and immobilization devices is one of the most severe types of pain that can be experienced.

   ❏ True   ❏ False

7. Upon application of a cast, a child should be informed that plaster generates coolness and that he or she should be prepared for the cast to feel cool.

   ❏ True   ❏ False

8. Osteomyelitis is most common in children between the ages of 16 and 18.

   ❏ True   ❏ False

9. Antibiotic therapy treatment for osteomyelitis most often lasts for one week.

   ❏ True   ❏ False

10. Developmental dysplasia of the hip is a term used to describe the condition in which the femoral head has an abnormal relationship to the acetabulum.

    ❏ True   ❏ False

11. Scoliosis is most often detected in children between 6 and 8 years of age.

    ❏ True   ❏ False

12. Osteogenesis imperfecta is a connective tissue disorder of the bones characterized by disturbed formation of periosteal bone.

    ❏ True   ❏ False

13. Compartment syndrome occurs when there is decreased pressure within a muscle compartment.

    ❏ True   ❏ False

14. Children who are immobilized are at risk for hypercalcemia because of bone demineralization.

    ❏ True   ❏ False

Fill in the Blank

1. The _____ is the shaft of the long bone, the _____ refers to the proximal and distal ends of the long bone, and the _____ is a section of the long bone in which the diaphysis and epiphysis converge and is responsible for growth until the child's adult height is attained.

2. Bone growth occurs in two ways: _____, or bone formation by osteoblasts, and _____, or resorption of old bony tissue.

3. The thin layer of cartilage located between the metaphysis and the epiphysis at the end of the long bones is called the _____.

4. The sports that have the highest risk of spine injury are _____, _____, _____, and _____.

5. Placement of children on a team is best determined by several factors, including _____, _____, _____, _____, and _____.

6. Initial treatment of sprains, strains, and contusions includes a treatment plan described by the acronym RICE: R_____, I_____, C_____, and E_____.

7. _____ traction is characterized by the child being in the supine position with both legs flexed slightly less than 90 degrees and the buttock off the mattress, whereas _____ traction is similar to the above-stated traction except a sling is under the knee suspending the affected leg.

8. For treatment of an unstable fracture of displaced vertebrae in the cervical and high thoracic areas of the spine, _____ are most often used.

9. The type of traction that is most commonly used for complicated fractures of the femur is _____.

10. _____ is an acute, nonpurulent inflammation of the synovial membrane of a joint that occurs most commonly in the hip joint.

11. Most people with muscular dystrophy die from _____ or _____ complications in their early_____ or late_____.

12. _____ is an excessive concave curvature of the lumbar spine.

Matching

_____ 1. greenstick fracture

_____ 2. strain

_____ 3. scoliosis

_____ 4. ecchymosis

_____ 5. crepitus

_____ 6. sprain

_____ 7. dislocation

_____ 8. oblique fracture

_____ 9. kyphosis

a. excessive concave curvature of the lumbar spine

b. stretching or tearing of a ligament

c. displacement of two bone ends or of a bone from its articulation with a joint

d. fracture line slanting or on a diagonal across the bone

e. humpback or rounded back deformity

f. talipes equinovarus

g. break through the periosteum and bone on one side while the other side only bends, resulting in an incomplete fracture

h. lateral curvature of the spine

i. stretching or tearing of either a muscle or tendon from overuse, overstretching, or misuse

_____ 10. subluxation

_____ 11. clubfoot

_____ 12. transverse fracture

_____ 13. lordosis

_____ 14. Legg-Calvé-Perthes

j. fracture line at right angles to the long axis of the bone

k. black and blue discoloration of an area of the skin

l. incomplete or partial dislocation of the articular surfaces of a joint

m. grating sound heard on the movement of the ends of a broken bone

n. osteochondrosis

Multiple Choice

1. A new nurse is caring for a child with a soft tissue injury. Which action by the new nurse requires the supervising nurse to intervene? The new nurse:

   a. elevates the affected limb to reduce swelling
   b. wraps the affected area with elastic wraps to avoid impaired neurovascular status
   c. uses narcotics to decrease severe pain associated with soft tissue injury
   d. restricts activity as necessary

2. In which phase of healing of the fracture does the callus turn into bone, the gap in the bone is bridged, and union occurs?

   a. inflammatory stage
   b. reparative stage
   c. ossification stage
   d. remodeling stage

3. Which of the following statements about traction is true?

   a. Traction is the application of pulling force to a body part against a countertraction pull exerted in the opposite direction.
   b. The process is used only to treat long bone fractures.
   c. Skin traction has a high risk of infection due to needed breakdown of the skin barrier.
   d. Traction causes muscle spasms and should be avoided in those types of fractures where muscle spasms are a common complication.

4. When working with a child who has sustained a fracture, the nurse identifies which as the least likely complication to occur?

   a. malunion

   b. infection

   c. compartment syndrome

   d. growth disturbance

5. Which of the following statements about cast removal in children is true?

   a. The pain most children feel is of moderate severity.

   b. Caregivers should be asked to remain out of the treatment area when the cast is being removed so the child can stay focused on the procedure.

   c. Yellow or brown flaking skin found under the removed cast area indicates an infection of the area has occurred.

   d. Instruct the caregivers to wash the extremity with warm water and a mild soap after the cast is removed.

6. Susan and Eric are Amy's parents. Amy fell from a counter she had crawled onto and sustained a fracture of her femur. Amy has been in Buck's traction for one week and will continue to be immobilized for at least five more weeks. Susan asks the nurse, "I don't know what has happened to Amy. She was such a sweet little girl. She is miserable. Will she ever be the same again?" The best response by the nurse is:

   a. To help Amy cope with her anger, fear, and immobility, use therapeutic touch, guided imagery, and humor.

   b. Tell your relatives to stay at home and not visit Amy until she is out of traction. This will be the most effective way to keep her calm.

   c. It is not normal for a child of Amy's age to experience a change of temperament due to immobilization. There must be something really wrong with her.

   d. The regressive behaviors Amy exhibits will stay with her.

7. Tatiana's child has clubfoot. She asks the nurse what kind of treatment she can expect her daughter to go through. The best response by the nurse is:

   a. Treatment will begin when your daughter is about 6 months old.

   b. It usually requires about one year of treatment to resolve the problem.

   c. There is no formal treatment; clubfoot resolves spontaneously.

   d. When serial casting is used as the method of treatment, the cast is changed every one to two weeks until complete correction has occurred.

8. Of the following, which is the priority nursing intervention for the child with Duchenne's muscular dystrophy?

    a. nutritional status
    b. genetic counseling
    c. respiratory status
    d. renal status

9. The nurse identifies all but which one of the following children as having a bone fracture as a result of physical abuse?

    a. Magda, age 4, who has a fracture of the tibia in different stages of healing
    b. Eli, age 7, who has a fracture of the sternum
    c. Jaoquine, age 2, who accidentally fell down the stairs and has a fracture of the ulna
    d. Yolanda, age 9 months, who has a fracture of the femur

10. The last physiologic process the body undergoes after a fracture is:

    a. inflammation
    b. reparative
    c. ossification
    d. remodeling

11. Which statement by a caregiver who will be providing care for a child with a newly applied cast indicates that more teaching is needed?

    a. The cast will be dry in 12 hours.
    b. I will handle the cast with the palm of my hand
    c. If my child experiences an itchy sensation under the cast. I will use a hair dryer on cool to blow air onto the itchy area.
    d. I will not allow the cast to become wet.

12. Which statement by the caregiver of a child with Legg-Calvé-Perthes Disease indicates that more teaching is needed?

    a. I will not allow my child to bear weight on the affected extremity.
    b. I will maintain my child on bedrest.
    c. I will maintain my child in adduction.
    d. This condition is caused by decreased blood supply to the femur bone.

Multiple Response

1. When working with children who have musculoskeletal injuries, it is important for the nurse to remember that which of the following statements about the differences between the child's and the adult's musculoskeletal system are true? Select all that apply.

   a. The bones of children contain large amounts of cartilage.
   b. The periosteum of children's bones is stronger and tougher with more osteogenic potential.
   c. Fractures occur more commonly in children than in adults.
   d. The bones of children are more porous.
   e. Children's bones are not able to bend.
   f. The periosteum of a child's bones is less vascular than an adult's.

2. Nursing management immediately following a musculoskeletal injury includes which of the following? Select all that apply.

   a. immobilization
   b. assessment of the neurovascular status of the affected extremity every 12 hours during the first 24 hours after injury
   c. assessment of skin color of the affected extremity
   d. assessment of skin temperature of the affected extremity
   e. assessment of pain
   f. assessment of pulses in the affected extremity

3. Nursing management for the child in traction includes which of the following interventions? Select all that apply.

   a. Be sure all weights are hanging freely.
   b. Maintain alignment.
   c. Assess the affected extremity for edema.
   d. Position the child's body to rest against the foot of the bed or the side of the bed.
   e. Remove the traction every 8 hours to perform range of motion.
   f. Provide pin care once a day.

4. Which of the following findings are strongly suggestive of abuse in the child? Select all that apply.

   a. multiple or depressed skull fractures
   b. frequent ear infections
   c. multiple fractures in various stages of healing
   d. spiral fracture of the humerus
   e. delayed mobility
   f. colic

5. Which of the following statements about Duchenne's muscular dystrophy are true? Select all that apply.

   a. Duchenne's muscular dystrophy affects girls more than boys.
   b. In children with Duchenne's muscular dystrophy, the calves appear large and strong, but in actuality they are weak because of infiltration of the muscles with fat and connective tissue.
   c. Most deaths from Duchenne's muscular dystrophy are due to respiratory infections or cardiac failure.
   d. There is no cure for Duchenne's muscular dystrophy.
   e. Children with Duchenne's muscular dystrophy usually walk on the tips of their toes.
   f. The father carries the gene for this disorder.

Critical Thinking/Case Study

George is a 9-year-old boy who sustained a greenstick fracture of his lower femur while riding a scooter. He is in 4th grade at a local school and has two older brothers. He lives in the same home with the other children and shares a bedroom with one of his brothers. Both the bedroom and bathroom are located on the second floor of the home. George has practiced all summer to be able to play football this year. George has a cast extending from his foot to his upper thigh.

1. List some possible nursing diagnoses for George based on NANDA.

   _____

   _____

   _____

2. George's father asks what a greenstick fracture is. How does the nurse reply?

   _____

   _____

   _____

3. Explain the healing process of a fracture by the four different stages.

   _____

   _____

   _____

4. What are the common complications of fractures of the long bones in children? What assessments should the nurse make to detect these complications? What interventions can the nurse incorporate into the plan of care to prevent the complications?

   _____

   _____

   _____

5. Develop a home care plan for George in relation to his cast.

   _____

   _____

   _____

CHAPTER 35

Psychosocial Alterations

True or False

1. Children with mental health problems are one of the most underserved populations in the health care system.

   ❑ True   ❑ False

2. Children and adolescents with psychosocial alterations or disorders are primarily treated in institutional settings.

   ❑ True   ❑ False

3. The goal of family therapy is to change family interactions, improve communications, and help family members achieve autonomy, independence, and self-effectiveness.

   ❑ True   ❑ False

4. Art therapy is used to assist the child to express feelings and issues difficult to verbalize.

   ❑ True   ❑ False

5. No one test or instrument is able to diagnose a child as having ADHD.

   ❑ True   ❑ False

6. Children with ADHD do not fall under the Education for All Handicapped Children Act; therefore, they do not receive free public education in the least restrictive environment.

   ❑ True   ❑ False

7. Children taking stimulant medications for ADHD will not become addicted to the medications.

   ❑ True   ❑ False

8. Mood disorders, also referred to as depressive disorders, are uncommon among children and adolescents.

   ❑ True   ❑ False

9. Biological theory proposes that the lack or excess of one or more neurotransmitters, specifically dopamine, may contribute to the development of depression.

   ❑ True   ❑ False

10. Compared to depressed adults, depressed children are often irritable, are more likely to express symptoms of anxiety, and have more somatic complaints such as stomachaches and headaches.

    ❑ True   ❑ False

11. Group therapy for children with depression is most effective if children in the group have the same diagnosis.

    ❑ True   ❑ False

12. Prevention programs for substance abuse may begin as early as elementary school and include education, peer teaching, and family involvement.

    ❑ True   ❑ False

13. In an individual with anorexia nervosa, weight should not be regained too quickly, as that is medically unsafe and may lead to cardiac overload and death.

    ❑ True   ❑ False

14. Strattera has not been found to have risks of abuse associated with its use.

    ❑ True   ❑ False

15. Asking a person about possible plans to commit suicide has been found to precipitate suicidal behavior.

    ❑ True   ❑ False

Fill in the Blank

1. Etiology of ADHD is unknown, but the following factors have been suggested: _____, _____, _____, and _____.

2. A deficiency in the neurotransmitter _____ has also been implicated in ADHD.

3. Stimulant medications used to treat ADHD increase the availability of _____ and _____ in the neural synapses, thus improving concentration and attention and reducing the child's activity level.

4. Depressive disorders are characterized by a pervasive mood disturbance involving _____, _____, _____, _____, _____, and _____.

5. Separation anxiety is a part of normal development from the age of _____ through _____.

6. _____ is a maladaptive pattern of the use of alcohol or drugs leading to significant distress or impairment.

7. Eating disorders such as _____ and _____ are common disorders encountered in children, especially adolescents.

8. Cardiovascular symptoms in the individual with bulimia may include _____, _____, and _____.

9. The three subtypes of attention-deficit hyperactivity disorder include _____, _____, and _____.

10. _____ is the first nonstimulant drug approved by the FDA for the treatment of attention-deficit hyperactivity disorder.

Matching

_____ 1. methylenedioxymethamphetamine

_____ 2. imipramine

_____ 3. fluoxetine

_____ 4. anhedonia

_____ 5. amitriptyline

a. marked decreased interest or pleasure in previously enjoyed activities

b. Tofranil

c. Elavil

d. Prozac

e. Ecstasy

Multiple Choice

1. An older teenager is undergoing individual therapy for a psychosocial issue. Which action by the new nurse providing the therapy will require the supervising nurse to intervene? The new nurse says:

   a. the teen that he or she can deny their caregivers access to their records

   b. the therapist and the child determine what will be shared with the caregivers

   c. caregivers will not take part in the session during individual therapy

   d. caregivers have no role in a comprehensive treatment program

2. Juawana is 13 years old. She is in need of therapy. Which treatment modality is considered to be powerful and effective for her age group?

   a. individual therapy
   b. family therapy
   c. group therapy
   d. play therapy

3. Which of the following children would most likely not exhibit behaviors similar to those seen with ADHD?

   a. John, age 8, who is depressed
   b. Eva, age 6, who has frequent otitis media
   c. Raul, age 10, who has a diagnosed learning disability
   d. Sandra, age 9, who is a juvenile diabetic

4. Which one of the following statements by a student nurse indicates that more teaching is needed? The diagnostic criteria for attention-deficit hyperactivity disorder include:

   a. low IQ scores
   b. difficulty waiting for his or her turn
   c. excessive talking
   d. difficulty organizing tasks

5. A child has been ordered to receive stimulant medications for the treatment of attention-deficit hyperactivity disorder. Which of the following medication orders will the nurse question? The child has been ordered to receive:

   a. methylphenidate (Ritalin)
   b. fluoxetine HCL (Prozac)
   c. dextroamphetamine sulfate (Dexedrine)
   d. amphetamine mixed salts (Adderall)

6. Upon assessment of a teenager who has overdosed on amphetamines, the nurse would expect to find which one of the following?

   a. hyperthermia
   b. hypotension
   c. convulsions
   d. tachypnea

Multiple Response

1. A child is placed on a selective serotonin reuptake inhibitor for the treatment of depression. When teaching the caregiver about the medications, which of the following will the nurse include? Select all that apply.

   a. It will take about one week before your child will feel less depressed.
   b. Your child may experience agitation as a side effect of the medication.
   c. Common side effects of these medications include changes in appetite.
   d. Individuals taking these medications may develop insomnia.
   e. You can expect your child's urine to turn orange as a result of taking this medication.
   f. Once your child starts to feel better, the medication should be stopped.

2. The nurse has performed an assessment on Eduardo, age 14. He told the nurse he feels like killing himself. Which of the following are appropriate responses by the nurse? Select all that apply.

   a. How do you plan to kill yourself?
   b. You really don't want to do that. I can help you.
   c. Where do you plan to do it?
   d. Do you have what you need to carry the plan out?
   e. You are too strong of a person to do that.
   f. You can't do that to your family.

3. Which of the following assessment findings would the nurse expect to find in a client with bulimia nervosa? Select all that apply.

   a. erosion of tooth enamel
   b. increased dental caries
   c. tooth discoloration
   d. hypertension
   e. irregular heart beat
   f. generalized muscle hypertrophy

Critical Thinking/Case Study

A pediatric nurse practitioner (PNP) specializing in treatment of children with attention-deficit hyperactivity disorder (ADHD) is preparing to provide a talk to parents of a local parent-teacher association.

1. What type of information should the PNP cover regarding the incidence and etiology of this disorder?

    _____

    _____

    _____

2. How should the PNP describe the relationship of dopamine to ADHD?

    _____

    _____

    _____

3. One of the parents asks, "How can you definitely tell that my child does or does not have ADHD?" How could the PNP best respond?

    _____

    _____

    _____

4. What would be the most effective method for the PNP to use in explaining pharmaco-therapy of ADHD?

    _____

    _____

    _____

5. How should the PNP summarize behavior management, educational interventions, and family education for the child with ADHD?

    _____

    _____

    _____

6. One of the participants asks, "When will my daughter outgrow ADHD?" How should the PNP respond?

_____

_____

_____

7. What services are available for children with ADHD?

_____

_____

_____

8. What type of structure should the caregivers use in the home setting for the child with ADHD?

_____

_____

_____

CHAPTER 36

Child Abuse and Neglect

True or False

1. Some folk medicine practices resemble child abuse.

   ❑ True   ❑ False

2. Caregivers who abuse their children tend to be older.

   ❑ True   ❑ False

3. Most deaths from abuse are a result of neurologic injury to the child.

   ❑ True   ❑ False

4. Children with an intracranial bleed, retinal hemorrhage, and possible long bone fractures should be suspected of having shaken baby syndrome.

   ❑ True   ❑ False

5. Fractures are the second major cause of abuse-related death.

   ❑ True   ❑ False

6. Children who are neglected generally demonstrate extreme agitation and disattachment toward the caregiver.

   ❑ True   ❑ False

7. When sexual abuse is suspected, use of a Wood's lamp can help in identifying semen.

   ❑ True   ❑ False

8. Most states require nurses, physicians, school personnel, social workers, and law enforcement personnel to report suspicions of child abuse/neglect.

   ❑ True   ❑ False

9. In most states, those individuals reporting abuse in good faith are immune from any civil or criminal liability.

   ❑ True   ❑ False

Fill in the Blank

1. In the _____ model of family violence, child abuse and neglect are seen as isolated events in a family system, and family violence is a pattern of behavior that is passed from generation to generation.

2. The _____ suggests society contains the attitudes, values, and beliefs that legitimize violence in the family.

3. Some folk medicine practices that resemble abuse include _____, which involves rubbing a coin or spoon heated in oil on an ill child's neck, spine, and ribs, and _____, which involves creating a vacuum under a cup or glass when a small amount of burning material is placed on the skin.

4. A(n) _____ examination assists in confirming the diagnosis of shaken baby syndrome, since a classic sign is_____.

5. _____ is an unlawful, sudden, violent attack on another person; _____ is sexual intercourse between closely related persons; and _____ involves prostitution and child pornography.

6. Four factors that describe the experience of sexually abused children and the consequent effect the abuse has on their growth and development include: _____, _____, _____, and _____.

Matching

____ 1. physical abuse

____ 2. scald burn

____ 3. psychological abuse

____ 4. child maltreatment

____ 5. child abuse

____ 6. immersion burn

a. intentional injury of a child

b. burn with an even line across the legs, buttocks, or hands

c. range of intentional behaviors by a parent or caregiver that can involve neglect and/or physical, emotional, and sexual abuse

d. caused by hot water from the tap, coffee, tea, or hot cooking grease

e. bodily injury to a child that appears to have been inflicted by other than accidental means

f. burn with a zebra pattern

_____ 7. child neglect

g. habitual lack of attention to the child's needs; it includes lack of affection, emotional support, and supervision

_____ 8. flexion burn

h. harmful, malicious, or ignorant withholding of physical, nutritional and health care, or emotional and educational necessities that provide a foundation for healthy childhood development

Multiple Choice

1. Which of the following attachment patterns describes an infant who realizes the caregiver will not always be available to provide comfort, who exhibits independent behavior without acknowledging the caregiver prior to separation, exhibits minimal distress during separation, and avoids emotional support offered by the caregiver upon reunion?

   a. secure
   b. avoidant
   c. ambivalent
   d. disorganized

2. Bianca is a nurse working in the emergency department. She is evaluating a 3-year-old boy who has been brought to the hospital because his father said he fell down a flight of stairs. The child has bruising over most of his body. Bianca identifies those bruises that are yellow-brown and fading to have occurred how long ago?

   a. one to two days ago
   b. three to five days ago
   c. five to seven days ago
   d. over one week ago

3. Which of the following statements would the nurse include when providing an inservice to staff members on Munchausen syndrome?

   a. The mother usually injures the child.
   b. The child is really not sick so they should never be admitted to the health care facility.
   c. There have been no identified benefits for the caregiver of the child.
   d. Individuals with this disorder always have a self-inflated ego.

4. Physical indicators of sexual abuse in children include which of the following?

   a. insomnia

   b. delayed language development

   c. retinal hemorrhage

   d. positive VDRL

5. A caregiver of a child has received information on ways to protect children from sexual abuse. Which statement by the caregiver indicates that more education is needed?

   a. Do not allow children to play unsupervised or in bedrooms with the door shut.

   b. Teach the child to tell a trusted caregiver or a teacher immediately if anyone touches him or her inappropriately.

   c. Insist that children have respect for adults and do everything they are told to do without question.

   d. Teach children to shake hands with others so they feel safer.

Multiple Response

1. Which of the following statements about Mongolian spots are true? Select all that apply.

   a. They are most commonly found on the chest.

   b. They are also referred to as birthmarks.

   c. They will not fade.

   d. They will remain stable over time.

   e. They are exclusively found in individuals of Asian decent.

   f. They require surgical removal.

2. Which of the following statements about shaken baby syndrome are true? Select all that apply.

   a. It is usually found in children under 3 years of age.

   b. Subdural hematomas of the brain are often found.

   c. The infant often has marks around the legs where he or she has been held and shaken.

   d. Infants and children with hypothermia should be suspected of possibly having shaken baby syndrome.

   e. Retinal hemorrhages are often found.

   f. Aortic aneurysms are a frequent finding.

3. Which of the following children would be considered a victim of psychological abuse? Select all that apply.

   a. Danesh, whose caregivers willfully did not attend his graduation ceremony from kindergarten

   b. Ophelia, age 12, whose mother tells her that her acne makes her look ugly

   c. Jamal, who is told by his father that he was a mistake

   d. Jorge, who is not fed any food for the day because he did not take a nap the day before

   e. Amelia, who is made to stay in wet clothes because she did not make it to the potty on time

   f. Jansen, who has to sit on the steps for 4 hours because he hit his younger sister

Critical Thinking/Case Study

Sophia, age 10, is seen in the primary care office. Her mother complains that Sophia, who used to be an excellent student, is having learning problems and failing grades. Sophia's mother tells the nurse, "She was such a happy child. Now she has a hard time sleeping; she seems very sad and quiet. Sophia has nightmares and is very upset and hostile when I ask her what's wrong. I want you to tell me what is going on with her because she is not the daughter I once knew." Sophia has not told her mother that she has been sexually abused by her 17-year-old stepbrother who has recently moved into their home.

1. What types of questions should the nurse ask to further assess this situation?

   _____

   _____

   _____

2. Which pieces of information given by the mother would lead the nurse to suspect sexual abuse as a cause of the change in Sophia's behavior?

   _____

   _____

   _____

3. What physical indicators of sexual abuse would the nurse expect to find?

_____

_____

_____

4. Why do you think Sophia has not told her mother about the sexual abuse by her stepbrother?

_____

_____

_____

Answers

CHAPTER 1: OVERVIEW OF PEDIATRIC NURSING

True or False

1. False
2. True
3. True
4. True
5. True
6. True
7. True

Fill in the Blank

1. low wages for women, low educational attainment of many single mothers, low rates and levels of child support from fathers
2. upper respiratory, ear, and skin infections; diarrhea; infestations (scabies and lice)
3. physical activity, overweight and obesity, tobacco use, substance abuse, responsible sexual behavior, mental health, injury and violence, environmental quality, immunizations, access to health care
4. 2,500 grams (5 pounds, 8 ounces)
5. education, environment and product changes, legislation or regulation
6. injury from farm machinery, pesticide exposure
7. atraumatic care

Matching

1. c
2. b
3. a

Multiple Choice

1. a
2. c
3. d

Multiple Response

1. a, b, d
2. b, c, d, e, f
3. a, c, d, e, f

CHAPTER 2: LEGAL AND ETHICAL ISSUES

True or False

1. False
2. True
3. True
4. False
5. False
6. False
7. True
8. False
9. True
10. True

Fill in the Blank

1. Informed consent

2. Assent

3. minor

4. medical forensic examination

5. Bioethics

6. Emancipation

7. passive euthanasia

8. age of majority

Matching

1. e

2. a

3. d

4. c

5. b

6. h

7. g

8. f

Multiple Choice

1. c

2. b

3. d

4. c

5. a

6. a

7. a

Multiple Response

1. b, c, d

2. a, c, d, f

3. a, b, c

4. a, c, d

CHAPTER 3: THE CHILD IN CONTEXT OF THE FAMILY

True or False

1. True

2. False

3. False

4. True

5. False

6. True

7. False

8. True

9. True

10. True

Fill in the Blank

1. family

2. Newman

3. Roy

4. affective, socialization and social placement, reproductive, economic, health care

5. Primary prevention

6. Cultural sensitivity

7. extended

8. blended family, stepfamily

Matching

1. c

2. a

3. c

4. b

5. d

Multiple Choice

1. c

2. b

3. d

4. a

Multiple Response

1. a, c, d

2. a, b, d

3. c, d, e, f

CHAPTER 4: COMMUNITY AND HOME HEALTH NURSING

True or False

1. True
2. False
3. True
4. True
5. True
6. False
7. False
8. True
9. False
10. True

Fill in the Blank

1. clinician, advocate, collaborator, consultant, counselor, educator, researcher, case manager
2. Health promotion
3. Health protection
4. Disease prevention
5. Tertiary prevention
6. Respite care

Matching

1. d
2. b
3. c
4. a

Multiple Choice

1. d
2. c
3. b
4. d
5. a

Multiple Response

1. a, c, d
2. b, c, d
3. a, b, d

CHAPTER 5: SCHOOL NURSING

True or False

1. False
2. False
3. True
4. True
5. False
6. True
7. False
8. True
9. True
10. True

Fill in the Blank

1. Direct service, indirect service
2. transmission, susceptibility, favorable environment
3. Hand washing
4. strep throat, scabies, lice
5. Type 2 diabetes, hypertension, high cholesterol
6. individual health plan (IHP)
7. sniffing, huffing
8. awareness

Matching

1. c
2. d
3. e
4. a
5. b

Multiple Choice

1. c
2. c
3. b
4. c

Multiple Response

1. b, c, d, e
2. a, b, d, e
3. b, c, d, e
4. a, b, c, e
5. b, d, e
6. a, b, c, d, e

CHAPTER 6: THEORETICAL APPROACHES TO THE GROWTH AND DEVELOPMENT OF CHILDREN

True or False

1. False
2. True
3. False
4. False
5. True
6. False
7. True
8. True
9. True
10. True

Fill in the Blank

1. Nature
2. Continuity
3. critical period
4. psychosexual
5. sex
6. Erickson
7. oral, trust versus mistrust, sensorimotor
8. interpersonal relations, basic needs

9. schema
10. inclusiveness, consistency, accuracy, relevance, fruitfulness, simplicity

Matching

1. i
2. a
3. j
4. k
5. l
6. c
7. f
8. b
9. g
10. d
11. e
12. h

Multiple Choice

1. a
2. d
3. d
4. c
5. b
6. a
7. c

Multiple Response

1. a, b, d, e
2. a, c, d, e
3. b, c, d

CHAPTER 7: GROWTH AND DEVELOPMENT OF THE NEWBORN

True or False

1. True
2. True
3. False

4. True

5. True

6. False

7. True

8. False

Fill in the Blank

1. 28 days or 4 weeks

2. placenta, umbilical arteries and veins, ductus venosus, foramen ovale, ductus arteriosus

3. caput succedaneum, cephalohematoma

4. 3, 8–18

5. 100, 150

6. Kernicterus

7. brown adipose tissue

8. Phototherapy

9. milia, petechiae, Mongolian spot

10. Spina bifida

11. talipes deformity

12. a relatively large body surface area, poor thermal insulation, limited shivering response, increased metabolic rate

13. pillows, comforters, blankets, sheepskins

Matching

1. c

2. d

3. a

4. e

5. b

Multiple Choice

1. a

2. c

3. d

4. b

5. c

6. d

7. a

Multiple Response

1. b, c, d, f

2. a, c, d, f

3. a, b, d

CHAPTER 8: GROWTH AND DEVELOPMENT OF THE INFANT

True or False

1. False

2. False

3. True

4. False

5. True

6. True

7. False

8. False

9. True

10. True

11. True

12. True

Fill in the Blank

1. 2 months of age, 12 to 18 months of age

2. maintain balance, exhibit posture control, initiate locomotion

3. 6 to 7

4. 2, 4, 6, 9

5. 7, 10

6. deciduous, primary, baby

7. low-grade fever, vomiting, diarrhea, mild abdominal pain

8. iron-fortified rice cereal

9. cow's milk

10. Colic

Matching

1. c
2. e
3. b
4. d
5. a

Multiple Choice

1. b
2. c
3. d
4. c
5. d
6. b
7. c
8. a
9. c
10. a
11. c

Multiple Response

1. b, c, d, e
2. b, c, d, e, f
3. a, c, d
4. b, c, d, e

CHAPTER 9: GROWTH AND DEVELOPMENT OF THE TODDLER

True or False

1. False
2. True
3. False
4. True
5. True
6. False
7. True
8. True
9. False
10. True
11. False
12. True

Fill in the Blank

1. physiologic anorexia
2. gaining self-control, developing autonomy, increasing independence
3. ritualism
4. Temper tantrums
5. 18–24
6. parallel play
7. pieces of hot dogs, nuts, hard candy
8. Mylar (foil-type)
9. Sibling rivalry
10. Temper tantrums

Matching

1. b
2. c
3. a

Multiple Choice

1. c
2. d
3. a
4. b
5. c
6. d
7. c
8. c
9. a
10. d

Multiple Response

1. a, b, d
2. b, c, d
3. a, b, d
4. c, e, f

CHAPTER 10: GROWTH AND DEVELOPMENT OF THE PRESCHOOLER

True or False

1. False
2. True
3. True
4. True
5. True
6. True

Fill in the Blank

1. Cognitive ability
2. preoperational
3. Oedipal, phallic
4. telegraphic, 3
5. superego
6. preconventional, premoral
7. one, two

Matching

1. c
2. d
3. a
4. b
5. e

Multiple Choice

1. c
2. d
3. b
4. c

Multiple Response

1. a, b, c
2. a, c, d, e
3. b, c, d
4. a, c, d

CHAPTER 11: GROWTH AND DEVELOPMENT OF THE SCHOOL-AGE CHILD

True or False

1. True
2. True
3. True
4. False
5. True
6. True
7. False
8. True
9. True
10. True

Fill in the Blank

1. balancing, catching, throwing, running, jumping, climbing
2. 90 to 95, 20
3. 8–13 and 10–14
4. latency
5. industry, inferiority
6. somnambulism
7. somniloquy
8. bullying

Matching

1. c
2. d
3. a
4. b

Multiple Choice

1. c
2. d
3. d
4. a

Multiple Response

1. a, b, c, e, f
2. b, c, d
3. c, e, f
4. a, c, d, e, f

CHAPTER 12: GROWTH AND DEVELOPMENT OF THE ADOLESCENT

True or False

1. True
2. True
3. False
4. True
5. False
6. False
7. True
8. True
9. False
10. True
11. True
12. True
13. True
14. True

Fill in the Blank

1. prepubertal (early), pubertal (middle), and postpubertal (late adolescence)
2. Puberty, Adolescence
3. somatropin
4. 12–14, 3–6, 4–10, 2½–5
5. enlargement/darkening of the nipple, growth/development, pubic, axillary
6. sperm production, maturation of seminiferous tubules, testicular maturation, testosterone
7. menarche
8. gynecomastia
9. egocentrism
10. "Who am I?", "What is my unique place in the world?"
11. friendship dyad, clique, the crowd
12. obesity, anorexia nervosa, bulimia nervosa
13. declining amounts of work-related and spontaneous physical activity; increased consumption of energy-dense, high-fat food; home environment itself
14. hepatitis, pancreatitis, gastritis, neuritis, cirrhosis, ulcers of the gastrointestinal tract, impotence, esophageal varices, cancer, cerebellar degeneration, delirium tremens, birth defects

Matching

1. d
2. a
3. f
4. b
5. c
6. i
7. e
8. h
9. g

Multiple Choice

1. c
2. c
3. d
4. a
5. b
6. a
7. a
8. c
9. b

Multiple Response

1. a, c, d, e, f
2. a, b, c, d, e
3. a, b, d, e, f

CHAPTER 13: CHILD AND FAMILY COMMUNICATION

True or False

1. True
2. True
3. False
4. True
5. False
6. True
7. True
8. True
9. True
10. False

Fill in the Blank

1. sender, message, channel, receiver, feedback
2. physical space or distance between receiver and sender, temperature or ventilation of the environment, distracting noise such as radios or television, health status (hearing or visual impairment), medical terminology, hearing or speech difficulties
3. personal judgments, past experience, emotions, developmental level, social values, perceived power differences of the sender and the receiver
4. Formal communication, Informal communication
5. tone and pitch of the voice, volume, inflection, speed, vocalization not considered language
6. establishing rapport, building trust, showing respect, conveying empathy, listening actively, providing appropriate feedback, managing conflict, establishing professional boundaries
7. Empathy
8. Be attentive, eliminate distractions; Be clear about the message, clarify if necessary; Be empathetic, convey concern and caring; Be open-minded, avoid prejudices

Matching

1. c
2. b
3. a

Multiple Choice

1. d
2. b
3. c
4. c
5. a
6. c
7. b
8. d

Multiple Response

1. b, c, d, e, f
2. a, c, d, e
3. b, c, d, e, f
4. a, c, d, e, f

CHAPTER 14: PEDIATRIC ASSESSMENT

True or False

1. True
2. True
3. False
4. False
5. True
6. False

7. True

8. True

9. False

10. False

11. True

12. False

13. True

14. True

15. True

16. True

Fill in the Blank

1. six

2. 24-hour food recall, food diary

3. serum albumin, prealbumin

4. anthropometric measurements

5. small for gestational age (SGA), 90th

6. setting sun sign

7. tip of the nose, external ear, lips, hands, feet

8. sudden painful cry during test, asymmetrical thigh skin folds, uneven knee level, limited hip abduction

9. cryptorchidism

10. inspection, auscultation, palpation

11. Denver 2

12. telangiectatic nevi

Matching

1. h

2. k

3. j

4. i

5. o

6. c

7. a

8. b

9. l

10. d

11. n

12. g

13. p

14. f

15. e

16. m

Multiple Choice

1. d

2. c

3. a

4. b

5. c

6. d

7. a

8. b

9. b

10. a

Multiple Response

1. b, c, d, e, f

2. b, c, d, e, f

CHAPTER 15: INFECTIOUS DISEASES

True or False

1. True

2. True

3. True

4. True

5. False

6. True

7. True

8. True

9. True

10. True

11. False

12. True

Fill in the Blank

1. antibiotics, specific immunizations
2. Infectious disease, Communicable disease
3. the microorganism, the method of transmission, the concentration of pathogens, the environment
4. infectious agent, reservoir, portal of exit, mode of transmission, portal of entry, susceptible host
5. vectors
6. Pneumococcus (streptococcus pneumoniae)
7. HIV
8. history of severe anaphylactic reaction to a vaccine or its component, encephalopathy within seven days of administration of DP/DtaP
9. prodrome
10. one to two, six

Matching

1. b
2. e
3. g
4. a
5. c
6. f
7. l
8. j
9. i
10. d
11. h

Multiple Choice

1. b
2. a
3. b
4. d
5. b

6. b
7. c
8. b
9. d

Multiple Response

1. b, c, d
2. d, e, f
3. a, e, f

CHAPTER 16: CARE OF CHILDREN WHO ARE HOSPITALIZED

True or False

1. True
2. True
3. True
4. False
5. False
6. True
7. False
8. True
9. False
10. True
11. False
12. True
13. False
14. True
15. True
16. True

Fill in the Blank

1. family, caregivers
2. Florence G. Blake
3. strength, growth
4. control, "hurt", separation
5. Atraumatic care
6. Therapeutic play
7. two to three
8. observation, manipulation

9. present

10. control, mastery

11. people are treated with dignity and respect; health care providers communicate and share complete and unbiased information with clients and families in ways that are affirming and useful; clients and family members build on their strengths by participating in experiences that enhance control and independence; and collaboration among clients, family members, and providers occurs in policy and program development and professional education, as well as in the delivery of care

12. protest, despair, denial

Matching

1. d

2. b

3. c

4. a

Multiple Choice

1. c

2. a

3. d

4. d

5. b

6. c

7. c

8. a

9. b

10. c

11. d

Multiple Response

1. a, c, d, e, f

2. b, c, d

3. a, b, d, e, f

4. a, b, c

CHAPTER 17: CHRONIC CONDITIONS

True or False

1. True

2. True

3. True

4. False

5. True

6. False

7. False

8. True

Fill in the Blank

1. Disability, handicap

2. marginality

3. Trajectory

4. accepting the condition, managing the condition, meeting the child's developmental needs, meeting the developmental needs of the family members, coping with stress and crisis, assisting family members to manage feelings, educating others about the condition, establishing a support system

5. Respite care

6. Ethnocentrism

Matching

1. b

2. f

3. a

4. g

5. c

6. d

7. e

Multiple Choice

1. d

2. b

3. a

4. c

Multiple Response

1. a, b, d

2. b, c, d

3. a, b, c, d

CHAPTER 18: PAIN MANAGEMENT

True or False

1. True

2. False

3. False

4. False

5. True

6. True

7. False

8. False

9. True

10. False

11. True

12. True

Fill in the Blank

1. analgesia

2. Acute pain, chronic pain

3. P—presence of pain: Are you hurting today?
   Q—quality: What words describe your pain (sharp, burning, and so on)?
   R—radiation/location: Where is your pain? Does it shoot or radiate anywhere else?
   S—severity: Give me a number between 0 and 10 for your pain.
   T—timing: How long have you had this pain? How long does it last when the pain comes?

4. Opioids

5. Morphine

6. Fentanyl

7. titration

8. Naloxone

9. aura

Matching

1. e

2. a

3. b

4. f

5. d

6. c

Multiple Choice

1. b

2. d

3. b

4. c

5. a

Multiple Response

1. b, c, d, e

2. a, b, c, e

3. a, b, d

CHAPTER 19: MEDICATION ADMINISTRATION

True or False

1. True

2. False

3. True

4. True

5. False

6. False

7. False

8. True

9. False

10. True

Fill in the Blank

1. Pharmacokinetics
2. slower, unreliable
3. Pharmacodynamics
4. right client, right medication, right dose, right route, right time, right documentation
5. urine, bile, sweat, saliva, expired air
6. kilogram, body surface area

Matching

1. d
2. a
3. c
4. b

Multiple Choice

1. a
2. b
3. d
4. a
5. b
6. a

Multiple Response

1. a, c, d, f
2. a, b, d
3. b, c, d
4. a, b, d

CHAPTER 20: LOSS AND BEREAVEMENT

True or False

1. True
2. True
3. False
4. True
5. True
6. True
7. True
8. True
9. True
10. True

Fill in the Blank

1. age, cognitive development
2. Parentification
3. universality, irreversibility, nonfunctionality, causality
4. Grief, bereavement, mourning
5. denial, anger, bargaining, depression, acceptance
6. to accept the reality of the loss, to experience the pain or emotional aspects of the loss, to adjust to an environment in which the deceased is missing, to relocate the dead person within one's life and find ways to memorialize the person

Matching

1. d
2. a
3. c
4. e
5. b

Multiple Choice

1. c
2. b
3. d
4. c
5. b
6. a
7. a
8. d
9. d

Multiple Response

1. a, b, d

2. b, c, d, e, f

3. a, b, d, e

CHAPTER 21: FLUID AND ELECTROLYTE ALTERATIONS

True or False

1. True

2. True

3. False

4. True

5. True

6. True

7. False

8. False

9. True

10. True

11. False

12. True

13. True

14. True

15. True

Fill in the Blank

1. percentage and distribution of body water, body surface area, rate of basal metabolism, status of kidney function

2. 10% glucose in water, dextrose 5% in ½ NS, dextrose 5% in RL

3. osmolarity

4. cardiac, ventricular fibrillation

5. Acidosis, alkalosis

6. hypotonic, isotonic, hypertonic

7. Acute gastroenteritis

8. bananas, rice, applesauce, tea or toast

9. thermal, electrical, chemical, radiation

10. eschar

11. Escharotomy

12. Debridement

13. homografts, heterografts

14. autograph

Matching

1. c

2. a

3. b

4. g

5. e

6. f

7. k

8. d

9. m

10. h

11. j

12. i

13. l

Multiple Choice

1. b

2. d

3. b

4. b

5. c

6. b

Multiple Response

1. a, c, d

2. a, b, d, e

3. b, c, d, e, f

CHAPTER 22: GENITOURINARY ALTERATIONS

True or False

1. False

2. True

3. False

4. False

5. True

6. True

7. False

8. True

9. True

10. True

11. False

12. True

13. True

Fill in the Blank

1. cystitis, pyelonephritis

2. Bladder exstrophy-epispadias complex

3. pyuria

4. enuresis

5. medications, bed-wetting alarms, motivational therapies, elimination diets, bowel programs for children who are constipated

6. carbonated beverages, dairy products, beverages with artificial coloring, citric fruit, heavily sugared foods, beverages with caffeine

7. Vesicoureteral reflux

8. Hypospadias

9. chordee, undescended testes, inguinal hernia

10. cryptorchidism, undescended testis

11. inguinal hernia, hydrocele

12. incarceration

13. proteinuria, hypoalbuminemia, edema, hyperlipidemia

14. acute renal failure, thrombocytopenia, anemia

Matching

1. d

2. j

3. c

4. e

5. h

6. f

7. b

8. k

9. i

10. g

11. a

12. l

Multiple Choice

1. c

2. a

3. a

4. b

5. d

6. c

Multiple Response

1. a, c, d

2. b, c, e

3. a, b, d, f

4. a, b, c

CHAPTER 23: GASTROINTESTINAL ALTERATIONS

True or False

1. False

2. True

3. True

4. True

5. False

6. False

7. False

8. True

9. True

10. True

11. True

12. True

Fill in the Blank

1. small, increased, increased

2. amylase, lactase

3. pyloromyotomy

4. nurse, plastic surgeon, neurosurgeon, ortho-
   dontist, otolaryngologist, pediatrician,
   speech pathologist, and audiologist

5. enlarge, stimulate, swallow, rest

6. Esophageal atresia

7. V—Verbal defect
   A—Anorectal malformation
   C—Cardiac defects
   T—Tracheoesophageal fistula
   E—Esophageal atresia
   R—Renal anomalies
   L—Limb defects

8. colicky, intermittent abdominal pain,
   vomiting, currant jelly-like stool

9. insufflation

10. P—Pain: front, back, side, and shoulders
    E—Electrolytes fall, shock ensues
    R—Rigidity or rebound of abdominal wall
    I—Immobility
    T—Tenderness
    O—Obstruction
    N—Nausea
    I—Increasing pulse, decreasing blood
    pressure
    T—Temperature falls, then rises
    I—Increasing girth of abdomen
    S—Silent abdomen

11. A, B, C

12. Intussusception

13. Hypertrophic pyloric stenosis

Matching

1. d

2. j

3. h

4. a

5. b

6. i

7. c

8. e

9. g

10. f

Multiple Choice

1. d

2. d

3. c

4. c

5. b

6. b

7. a

8. b

9. d

10. a

Multiple Response

1. a, b, c, e

2. b, c, d, e

3. b, c, e, f

4. c, d, e, f

CHAPTER 24: RESPIRATORY ALTERATIONS

True or False

1. True

2. False

3. True

4. True

5. False

6. True

7. True

8. True

9. True

10. False

11. True

12. True

13. True

14. False

15. False

16. True

17. True

18. True

19. True

20. False

Fill in the Blank

1. nasopharyngitis

2. scarlet fever, otitis media, suppurative infection of surrounding tissue

3. tympanoplasty

4. stridor

5. respiratory distress, fever, sore throat, dysphagia, drooling, agitation, and lethargy

6. expiratory wheezing, chronic cough, dyspnea

7. exocrine

8. bronchiectasis, pneumothorax, cor pulmonale

9. surfactant

10. bacillus of Calmette and Guerin (BCG)

11. periorbital cellulitis, osteomyletis, meningitis, brain abscess, cavernous sinus thrombosis

12. respiratory distress syndrome (RDS)

13. wheezing

14. controlling environmental hazards such as second-hand smoke, air pollution, allergens; minimizing the risk of infection through immunizations and infection control practices; genetic counseling; prenatal care; anticipatory guidance

15. community-acquired pneumonia

16. Ribavirin (Virazole)

Matching

1. c

2. a

3. e

4. b

5. d

Multiple Choice

1. b

2. a

3. c

4. a

5. d

6. d

7. b

8. b

9. a

10. a

11. c

12. c

Multiple Response

1. a, b, c

2. a

3. b, e, f

4. a, b, d, f

CHAPTER 25: CARDIOVASCULAR ALTERATIONS

True or False

1. True

2. False

3. False

4. False

5. True

6. True

7. True

8. True

9. False

10. False

11. True

12. True

13. False

14. True

15. True

16. False

17. True

18. True

19. True

20. True

Fill in the Blank

1. interruption of the umbilical cord, spontaneous respiration

2. Preload, Afterload

3. hypercyanosis

4. Clubbing

5. positive inotropes

6. indomethacin

7. DiGeorge syndrome

8. erythrocytosis

9. valvuloplasty, valvulotomy

10. ventricular septal defect, pulmonary stenosis, right ventricular hypertrophy, overriding aorta

11. aorta, pulmonary artery

12. upper extremity hypertension, arms and legs

13. warfarin (Coumadin)

14. Osler's nodes, Janeway lesions

15. renal

16. Supraventricular tachycardia

17. hypovolemic, distributive, cardiogenic

18. O negative (universal donor)

19. Captopril, Enalopril

Matching

1. l

2. i

3. j

4. k

5. d

6. a

7. e

8. c

9. b

10. f

11. h

12. g

Multiple Choice

1. c

2. d

3. a

4. b

5. d

6. b

7. a

8. c

9. d

10. b

Multiple Response

1. b, c, d

2. a, b, d

3. a, c, d, f

4. b, c, e

CHAPTER 26: HEMATOLOGICAL ALTERATIONS

True or False

1. True
2. True
3. True
4. True
5. False
6. True
7. True
8. True
9. True
10. False
11. True
12. False
13. True

Fill in the Blank

1. erythropoiesis, hemolysis
2. ferritin
3. ferrous
4. vaso-occlusive crisis
5. sequestration crisis
6. Thalassemia
7. hemosiderosis
8. chelating agent
9. hematomas
10. Pancytopenia
11. hemophilias
12. hemarthrosis

Matching

1. g
2. a
3. d
4. c
5. h
6. b
7. e
8. f

Multiple Choice

1. c
2. a
3. d
4. b
5. a
6. b
7. c
8. a
9. d
10. c

Multiple Response

1. a, c, d, e
2. a, b, d, e, f
3. b, c, d, e, f
4. b, c, d

CHAPTER 27: IMMUNOLOGIC ALTERATIONS

True or False

1. True
2. True
3. True
4. False
5. True
6. True
7. False
8. False
9. True
10. False
11. True
12. False
13. True
14. True

Fill in the Blank

1. autoimmunity
2. Acquired immunity
3. Passive immunity
4. AIDS
5. highly active antiretroviral therapy (HAART)
6. western blot
7. sulfamethoxazole/trimethoprim
8. Maculopapular

Matching

1. e
2. b
3. f
4. c
5. d
6. a
7. g

Multiple Choice

1. b
2. c
3. d
4. b
5. b
6. d
7. a

Multiple Response

1. a, b, d
2. a, b, d
3. b, c, d

CHAPTER 28: ENDOCRINE ALTERATIONS

True or False

1. True
2. True
3. False
4. True
5. True
6. False
7. True
8. False
9. False
10. False
11. False
12. True
13. True
14. False

Fill in the Blank

1. hormone
2. tropic hormones
3. protein, iodine
4. bone, kidney, gastrointestinal tract
5. high-pitched, increased fat, childlike with a large, prominent forehead, higher, height
6. depot injection
7. slipped femoral epiphysis, pseudotumor cerebri, edema, sodium retention
8. 7–8, 6–7, 9
9. Tanner staging
10. polyuria, polydipsia
11. cretinism
12. Graves' disease
13. Exophthalmos proptosis
14. virilization
15. pseudohermaphroditism
16. females

Matching

1. j
2. h
3. g
4. n
5. k

6. l

7. d

8. b

9. m

10. a

11. f

12. i

13. e

14. c

Multiple Choice

1. a

2. c

3. a

4. b

5. a

6. b

7. b

8. c

9. a

10. c

11. b

12. c

13. d

14. a

15. a

Multiple Response

1. a, b, c

2. a, c, d

3. a, b, d, e, f

4. a, b, c, e, f

5. a, b, d

CHAPTER 29: CELLULAR ALTERATIONS

True or False

1. False

2. False

3. True

4. False

5. True

6. True

7. False

8. True

9. False

10. False

11. True

12. False

13. True

14. True

15. False

16. True

Fill in the Blank

1. leukemia

2. Palliative

3. alkalating agents, antimetabolites, antitumor antibiotics, plant alkaloids, corticosteroids, miscellaneous agents

4. Handwashing

5. hemorrhagic cystitis

6. 48 hours, 5 days

7. colony stimulating factor (CSF), interleukins, monoclonal antibodies, interferon

8. Monoclonal antibodies

9. Interferon

10. tumor lysis syndrome

11. vesicants, extravasate

12. Brachytherapy

13. surgical resection

Matching

1. d

2. g

3. h

4. c

5. b

6. a

7. e

8. f

Multiple Choice

1. a

2. a

3. c

4. d

5. d

6. b

7. c

8. a

9. b

10. c

Multiple Response

1. a, c, d, e

2. a, b, d

3. a, b, c, e, f

4. b, c, d

5. d, e, f

CHAPTER 30: INTEGUMENTARY ALTERATIONS

True or False

1. True

2. False

3. True

4. True

5. True

6. True

7. False

8. False

9. False

10. True

11. True

12. False

13. True

14. False

15. False

16. True

17. True

18. False

19. True

20. False

Fill in the Blank

1. storage, absorption

2. Impetigo

3. erythema, swelling, warmth, pain

4. intertrigo

5. tinea capitis, tinea corporis, tinea pedis, tinea cruris, tinea unguium, onychomycosis

6. terbinafine (Lamisil)

7. 10

8. epinephrine

9. furuncle

10. melanin

11. retapamulin (Altabax)

Matching

1. h

2. f

3. k

4. a

5. j

6. i

7. c

8. e

9. d

10. b

11. l

12. g

Multiple Choice

1. d
2. d
3. b
4. d
5. a
6. a
7. b
8. b
9. d
10. a

Multiple Response

1. b, c, d, f
2. a, b, d, e, f
3. a, b, c, e
4. b, c, d, e, f

CHAPTER 31: SENSORY ALTERATIONS

True or False

1. True
2. True
3. True
4. False
5. True
6. False
7. False
8. True
9. False
10. True
11. True
12. True
13. True

Fill in the Blank

1. Speech
2. Stuttering

3. assessment, family education
4. Conductive hearing loss, Sensorineural hearing loss
5. decibel (dB), hertz (Hz)
6. Vibrotactile aids
7. Cued speech
8. Astigmatism
9. Strabismus
10. Amblyopia
11. 3

Matching

1. o
2. c
3. b
4. f
5. j
6. a
7. k
8. g
9. h
10. d
11. q
12. e
13. i
14. l
15. n
16. m
17. p

Multiple Choice

1. c
2. b
3. b
4. d
5. b
6. c
7. b

8. d

9. c

10. a

Multiple Response

1. b, c, d, e

2. a, b, d

3. b, c, e

4. a, c, d

CHAPTER 32: NEUROLOGICAL ALTERATIONS

True or False

1. True

2. True

3. False

4. False

5. True

6. True

7. True

8. False

9. False

10. True

11. True

12. False

13. False

14. True

15. True

Fill in the Blank

1. Decorticate, decerebrate

2. epileptogenic focus

3. Status epilepticus, Refractory, epilepsy

4. Rolandic or sylvian seizures, jacksonian seizures

5. ketogenic

6. Macewen's sign

7. folic acid

8. meningomyelocele, meningocele

9. alpha-fetoprotein

10. arteriovenous malformation

11. opisthotonic

12. Brudzinski sign, Kernig's sign

13. Coma

14. diazepam (Valium)

Matching

1. d

2. e

3. f

4. a

5. h

6. b

7. c

8. j

9. g

10. i

11. o

12. k

13. v

14. r

15. w

16. n

17. l

18. u

19. p

20. q

21. t

22. s

23. x

24. m

Multiple Choice

1. d

2. a

3. c

4. c

5. d

6. a

7. a

8. c

9. a

10. b

11. c

12. d

13. c

14. c

15. d

Multiple Response

1. a, b, c

2. b, c, e, f

3. b, c, d

4. a, b, c

5. b, c, f

CHAPTER 33: COGNITIVE ALTERATIONS

True or False

1. True

2. True

3. False

4. True

5. False

6. True

7. True

8. True

9. True

10. True

Fill in the Blank

1. Mental retardation

2. plasticity

3. denial, anxiety, fear, depression, guilt, anger

4. karyotyping

5. otitis media, mitral valve prolapse, gastroesophageal reflux

6. aberrant social skill development

7. cardiac defects, skeletal defects, ocular defects, renal anomalies

8. autism, Asperger's disorder/syndrome, childhood disintegrative disorder, Rett syndrome, pervasive developmental disorder not otherwise specified

Matching

1. e

2. d

3. b

4. g

5. h

6. c

7. a

8. f

Multiple Choice

1. c

2. b

3. a

4. d

5. a

Multiple Response

1. a, b, d

2. b, c, d, e

3. b, c, d, e

CHAPTER 34: MUSCULOSKELETAL ALTERATIONS

True or False

1. True

2. False

3. False

4. True

5. True

6. True

7. False

8. False

9. False

10. True

11. False

12. True

13. False

14. False

Fill in the Blank

1. diaphysis, epiphysis, metaphysis

2. osteoblastic activity, osteoclastic activity

3. epiphyseal growth plate

4. football, gymnastics, ice hockey, wrestling

5. age; size; and emotional, social, cognitive maturity

6. rest, ice, compression, elevation

7. Bryant's, Russell

8. Crutchfield tongs

9. 90/90 femoral traction

10. Synovitis

11. cardiac, respiratory, teens, twenties

12. Lordosis

Matching

1. g

2. i

3. h

4. k

5. m

6. b

7. c

8. d

9. e

10. l

11. f

12. j

13. a

14. n

Multiple Choice

1. c

2. c

3. a

4. b

5. d

6. a

7. d

8. c

9. c

10. d

11. a

12. c

Multiple Response

1. a, b, d

2. a, c, d, e, f

3. a, b, c

4. a, c, d

5. b, c, d, e

CHAPTER 35: PSYCHOSOCIAL ALTERATIONS

True or False

1. True

2. False

3. True

4. True

5. True

6. False

7. True

8. False

9. False

10. True

11. False

12. True

13. True

14. True

15. False

Fill in the Blank

1. genetic, neurophysiologic, dietary, environmental

2. dopamine

3. dopamine, norepinephrine

4. loss of interest or pleasure in normal activities, sadness, problems with sleep, appetite, energy, concentration

5. seven months, the preschool years

6. Substance abuse

7. anorexia nervosa, bulimia nervosa

8. hypotension, arrhythmias, cardiomyopathy

9. inattentive only, hyperactive impulsive, combined inattentive-hyperactive impulsive

10. Strattera

Matching

1. e

2. b

3. d

4. a

5. c

Multiple Choice

1. d

2. c

3. c

4. a

5. b

6. c

Multiple Response

1. b, c, d

2. a, c, d

3. a, b, c, e

CHAPTER 36: CHILD ABUSE AND NEGLECT

True or False

1. True

2. False

3. True

4. True

5. False

6. False

7. True

8. True

9. True

Fill in the Blank

1. sociological

2. social-interactional systemic perspective

3. Cao Gao, cupping

4. ophthalmologic, retinal hemorrhage

5. Assault, incest, exploitation

6. traumatic sexualization, stigmatization, betrayal, powerlessness

Matching

1. e

2. d

3. g

4. a

5. c

6. b

7. h

8. f

Multiple Choice

1. b

2. d

3. a

4. d

5. c

Multiple Response

1. b, c, d

2. a, b, d, e

3. a, b, c

CPSIA information can be obtained
at www.ICGtesting.com
Printed in the USA
FFOW03n0611130415
12564FF

9 781435 486706